SEX and QUANTUM PHYSICS

VOLUME 1:
Tantric Yogi Tells All

Paul Squassoni

SEX and QUANTUM PHYSICS
VOLUME 1: Tantric Yogi Tells All

Text and illustrations by Paul Squassoni

Copyright ©2011 BreatheDown Publishing.
All rights reserved.
ISBN # 978-0-9827184-1-4

BreatheDownPublishing
12-6860 Kalapana-Kapoho Road
Pahoa, HI 96778
www.SexandQuantumPhysics.com
books@breathedown.com

The best way to start is at the beginning...

Introduction

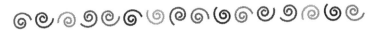

Sex and Quantum Physics. Just putting the words together brings a smile to the lips! What could possibly be farther apart? It conjures up images of sex in space, or in some weird quantum dimension.

In fact, there is no question that we live in a world that has both. Both the messiness of daily life with all its desires, emotions, thoughts and uncertainties, and also the elegant mathematical models of strange attractors, quantum foam, and multiple dimensions.

What kind of sense can we make out of living in a world that has both sex and quantum physics? We can begin by asking what sex and quantum physics have to say to each other.

Crazy?

Maybe. Maybe it takes the crazy wisdom of Tantra to weave the two into one cloth. But it doesn't really matter what you call it. What is much more important is how you live your life!

And putting sex and quantum physics together provides a remarkably useful set of tools for living richly and well.

You won't actually find much quantum physics in *Volume 1: Tantric Yogi Tells All*, though you will find dark energy and discoveries about the evolution of energy systems. And how they provide new ways of looking at everything from sex to human history.

Volume 1: Tantric Yogi Tells All is a story about almost everything. *Volume 2: Living in eleven dimensions* is the fun details: quantum physics, the nature of ecstatic insight, how to make your body really happy, and a much deeper discussion of sex and energy.

But to stay *pono* (a Hawaiian word for harmony) with the readers of this book, at the end is a topic from *Living in eleven dimensions* of how one discovery of quantum physics radically changes the way we understand the universe.

And make the idea of sex in a quantum dimension not only possible, but probable!

1 A Tantric teacup

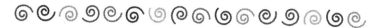

How would you like to start?

With a favorite Zen story...

A Cup of Tea

Nan-in, a Japanese master during the Meiji era (1868-1912), received a university professor who came to inquire about Zen. Nan-in served tea. He poured his visitor's cup full, and then kept on pouring.

The professor watched the overflow until he no longer could restrain himself. "It is overfull. No more will go in!"

"Like this cup," Nan-in said, "you are full of your own opinions and speculations. How can I show you Zen unless you first empty your cup?"

Why this particular story?

The meaning is very clear! You cannot begin to learn a new thing unless you approach it with a fresh mind. We have preconceptions about so many things... they act as filters that block our view of the very thing we are trying to see.

So we must empty our mind to see Tantra?

Not really, but we have to remember that we keep trying to fill the teacup with our own thoughts. We also need to make space, noticing our preconceptions and keeping them flexible enough to allow in new information.

To a Tantric, the teacup is not empty! It is filled with the same energy that flows through everything in the universe. There is room for our preconceptions, but also room for many new things besides. As we explore the teacup, our previous thoughts and experience interact with all the new things we find.

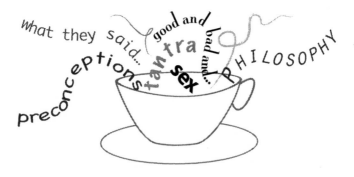

Isn't Tantra about sex?

That's a very full teacup you have! And a very common misconception. Tantra explores all of the energy centers, or chakras, of the body. We could talk about different representations of chakras (from seven to 36,000) for many days, but it is useful to stick with the seven everyone can find. One of them, the second, is associated with sexual energy. Tantra pays the same exquisite attention to the second chakra as it pays to all the others.

In short, Tantra is about everything, including sex. Because Tantra explores sexual energy as an aspect of life, it is much more strongly associated with sexual energy than other traditions.

What about all the "Tantric" workshops that explore sexual energy?

Supply and demand. The supply side are the people who begin to learn about Tantra and find such a sense of liberation when they explore their second chakra that they think: "This is it! Such freedom, such pleasure, such joy! I have found what I sought and this is what I will teach to others!"

They work with more than the second chakra, of course. They work with the heart, and the mind, and they use the second chakra to re-tune the other energy centers. All good work! But it is easy to become so focused on the second chakra that you do not continue to explore all your energy centers and learn how to integrate them.

The demand side is that there are a great many people in need of loosening up all the energy they buried in the second chakra over the course of their lives. This creates a ready market for what is often called "sexual healing." People look for this particular aspect of Tantra, they find it, and Tantra becomes reduced in the popular mind to a set of sexual techniques.

In truth, almost everything you can read about Tantric practices, including the most ancient texts, are complete nonsense!

Nonsense?

They are profoundly nonsensical, though many are beautiful poetry and succeed very well in describing different

states of being. Tantra pays exquisite attention to all of
the energy centers. How then can you take the experience
apprehended by seven (or 36,000) energy centers and reduce it
to words?

Words are a product of the mind and speech centers. They
are a marvelous invention and very, very useful! But it is not
possible to translate the experience and energy of your entire
body into something produced by two or three centers.

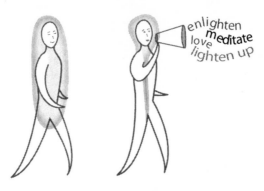

Why, then, were they written?

As explorers, we make maps so we can share with others
where we have been and where other people can go, too.

The words we use are a map pointing to a real experience,
but they are not the experience itself. Alfred Korzybyski, a
founder of general semantics, expressed this beautifully. He
said, *The map is not the territory.*

The maps, composed of words and images, songs and
religions, change with each culture. Almost all of them offer
great insights and beauty, teaching us new patterns and ways
of living. Some are very good maps, but they are still just
maps.

Don't mistake the map for the territory. You have to do the exploring yourself.

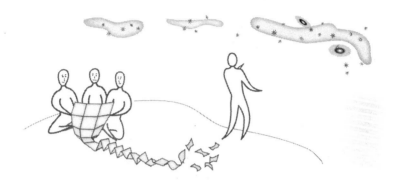

Is this book a new map?

In some ways, yes. The existing maps of Tantra and other traditions are beautiful and useful. The chants and exercises, colors, sounds and images, are all designed to evoke states of connectedness with the universe, which is all that matters. If it works, use it!

Mapmaking, however, takes place in a cultural context. An ancient map may show the world resting on the back of a turtle or elephant. A medieval map will show monsters past the flat edge of the world. The maps of each culture reflect the shared understanding of that culture as to the nature of the world.

We live in a new culture, the first global culture ever attempted by humans. Our map needs satellites and radio waves, evolution and an expanding universe. It needs chaos and organization, and a more sophisticated understanding of the ways humans live and interact.

To answer your question in another way, the words we are using will help create a modern context for an unfolding

experience of Tantra. They will be no more useful, and no
less, than ancient texts and all the beautiful images humans
have created. But they will hopefully be more to the point,
more tied to our modern understanding of the universe, and
verifiable in our own experience.

Verifiable? How?

Tantra is not mystical. It is not spiritual. It has nothing to
do with belief.

Tantra is practical and experiential. It is the enhanced
perception that occurs when you perceive with all of your
energy centers and not just one or two of them. It is what you
feel every day.

That's what makes it verifiable. Test your perception,
your perspectives, your experience of your own body, in the
exercises in this book. Test them in your everyday life. Explore
for yourself.

Oh... and don't mistake anything in these conversations
as truth. Truth is the name we give to assumptions, or
conclusions based on assumptions. Verify! Verify! Verify! Any
way you can! Take every sentence in this book as an invitation
to test it against your own experience.

No two people can have the exact same truth, though
we may agree on almost everything. Every single human is a
unique lens, with unique properties, and what each of us sees
of the universe is unique. Develop your own lens, and find
your own truth...

You mention the universe a lot...

Sometimes it seems that the hardest thing for humans to
do is accept that they live in the universe. We are in it, we are

of it: the universe is the warp and weft of our fabric, it is that which weaves us.

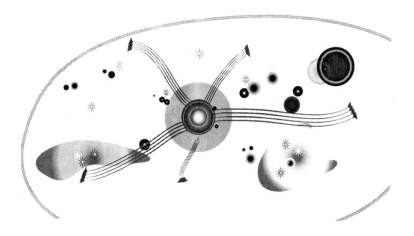

We come into this life and immediately begin to attach ourselves to all kinds of things: family, emotions, fears, friends, lovers, ideas, spirituality… we chop our experience of the universe into many pieces and chase whatever pieces we think we desire, when in fact our desire is to connect to the whole.

So far the word Tantra has been used here to mean different things: a tradition, a set of tools for exploration, the universe. Tantra at its root, though, means "weave," as in the fabric of the universe. As a tradition, it is *Mahamudra*, the Great Way that encompasses all other ways of exploration.

There are no rules in Tantra, because it is pure exploration of the universe. As we shall see, the universe is not something "other," not some vast, unimaginable void that has a corner seat we have been plunked into.

The universe is very much alive, or we could not be. Sometimes the word "universe" seems too cold to me, and I use the word "Goddess" instead. Use whatever word you like, there are no rules!

What's next?

Exploring! Exploring the body, exploring the energy in our bodies, the patterns of our lives, the patterns of humans, the patterns of the universe... there is no end to the exploration!

We'll play with releasing energy from the tension in our bodies, opening up the front and back of our bodies, discovering where in the body we put all our past experiences and emotions. We'll explore why our physical bodies are made of energy, how to work with that energy, and how that relates to the energy in everything else.

We'll have to talk a little about sparkling insights from physics and dark energy and thermodynamics, using the latest downloads from the universe as an explorer's map.

And if we explore, we'll begin to see why everything in the entire universe is unique, and why it is cherished. Why we are on the most exciting adventure we could possibly imagine: the evolution of the universe.

2 Breathe down

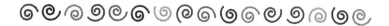

Without breath, there is no life. Without aware breath, our awareness is limited.

Oddly enough, breathing is so fundamental and so wired into us that few of us are ever actually taught how to breathe. We are told to take deep breaths when we are upset or angry. Children hold their breath to get what they want from their parents. And of course, athletes learn to time their breath with their exertions.

Working with the breath, known as *pranayama* in yoga, is important in many traditions. These traditions have discovered that the breath is so integral to awareness that you can change your state of awareness through focusing on and changing your breath.

From a Tantric point of view, the body already knows a lot about pranayama; we are already wired to change our breath as different frequencies of energy flow through us. Think of the sudden intake of breath when we are struck with wonder, or the almost cessation of breath when we are in a meditative trance. The heartfelt sigh releases tension in our heart and breath centers.

How is it we do this?

Most people think of breathing as an expansion and contraction of the lungs. That is not quite the whole picture. The lungs mostly exchange oxygen and carbon dioxide between the blood vessels in the lungs and the air in the chest cavity. Breathing is the expansion and contraction of the space inside the chest. While expanding the space can be done by moving the rib cage inwards and outwards, it is much more effective to change the size of the space using the diaphragm.

In the diagrams below, look at the how the diaphragm moves down to expand the chest space on the in-breath, and returns to a neutral position on the out-breath.

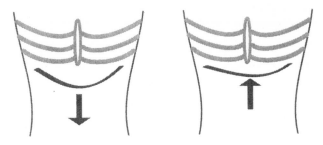

Now we can explore different ways to expand the chest space. The first diagram below shows a rib cage breath. The center diagram shows a belly breath, in which expanding the belly draws down the diaphragm. The third shows a pelvic breath, where all the muscles attached to the pelvis help pull down the diaphragm.

Try all three, experimenting with different muscles and positions. Focus on the in-breath and let the out-breath take care of itself. Deep breaths are not necessary. In fact, a gentler breath gives you more options and better control!

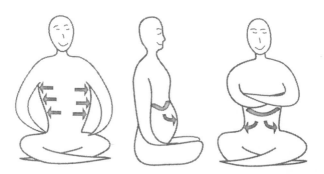

The type of breath you use changes for different activities. The chest breath will work fine for exploring breathing down.

Why *down*?

Natural orientation for humans seems to be up. Higher is better; the head is more sacred than the feet, and much prettier, too!

But the feet and the bottom of the spine are our connection to the ground, to gravity, which is merely one of the biggest forces in our lives.

Breathing "down" connects us to the ground, and opens up our base chakra. It's very simple.

- Seat yourself in a comfortable cross-legged position (or really, any position will do!).
- Take an easy, good breath.
- Focus the out-breath down through your body into the ground.

The air doesn't travel down, but it may well feel as though it does. Explore a couple breaths. You will know when you have breathed down. Your sit bones will drop closer to the floor, your spine will begin to straighten of its own accord, your head will move up and back so that it is more directly over the spine.

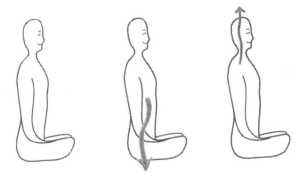

If you let the top of your head relax a bit, at the end of the down-breath you may even feel a little energy rise through the neck and out the top of the head.

Play with your breathing. You don't have to breathe down with every breath; on some breaths instead let your spine sway a little on the out-breath. Just remember at some point to breathe in, breathe down, pause, and THEN let yourself move again.

That's simple...

Such a simple thing, a simple thing that has no end to it! As you breathe down, you will notice that the rib cage relaxes, the heart settles to a gentler pace, the shoulders drop, the hips widen.

Try it sitting, standing, waiting for a bus or a train.

Hug someone and breathe down at the same time. You'll be amazed at the difference! Better yet, get them to breathe down with you during the hug. Just tell them "Breathe in, and breathe down through your feet into the ground." It will feel completely different from any hug you have ever encountered.

Why?

Breath is energy, and there is energy in the patterns of our breathing. There HAS to be, because we use the energy of our bodies to do it.

When you change the patterns of your breathing, you are changing the pattern of the energy that powers that breathing, the pattern that vibrates like a shell around you as your chest rises and falls.

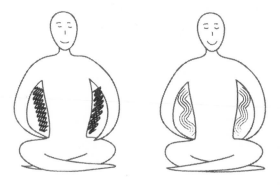

Relax the shell, let the energy patterns relax and gentle themselves, and you will be in a different energy state. If you are hugging someone at the same time, the change in state is even more pronounced.

Welcome to Tantric physics!

3 Your body is tensile!

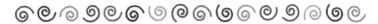

As the awareness of our breath tends to be uneducated, so too does the awareness of our bodies. Your body is more than a cart for carrying around your head!

Everyone knows that the body is made up of bones and muscles, and many know that it is all held together by connective tissue called fascia. Since our thinking still tends to be mechanical, very often we think of the body as a mechanical structure, in which the bones are levers and the muscles are pulleys. Like when you lift weights.

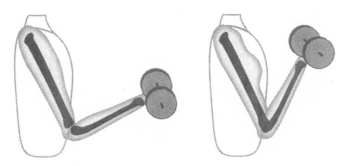

This is not incorrect when you consider the big muscles of the body, but the body is so much more than this. The body is a tensile structure, which means that it has tension, and that it can be stretched and drawn out. Not even our bones are fixed! Bones are made of millions of cells joined together and are designed to flex in three dimensions under pressure.

Our joints are not mechanical either, but composed of a dense web of connections that provide for stretching, twisting, flexing, lengthening and shortening. In fact, if you imagine the body as a computer simulation made up of thousands of lines all crisscrossing each other, you will have a better model of the body than our old mechanical picture.

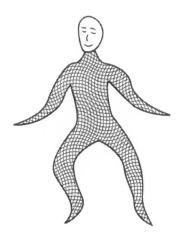

Why do visuals matter?

Because it is one of the most important ways we consciously explore and interact with our bodies. We certainly have wiring for basic movements dating back to our reptilian ancestry and genes, and many patterns in our bodies are automatic, or nearly so. But our conscious movements depend on our brains. If we see the arm as a lever and pulley, we will only move it as a lever and pulley. If we see it and move it as a tensile structure, which can move like a snake in three dimensions, our range of movement will be much greater.

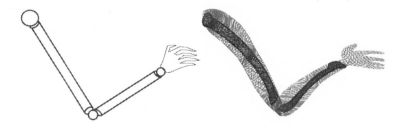

And if we see the body as a tensile structure...

We will have a more accurate map through which we can explore and use our bodies. And also a way to begin to make sense of the connection between our physical bodies and the energy locked into them.

Whoa! What are you saying?

The body is a tensile structure. It is under tension. If it were not, we would be formless blobs on the floor!

What is tension? Muscles contract because of a chemical bond between myosin and actin. When that bond is released, and the muscle relaxes, energy is released. The tighter the body, the more energy we are using to keep it that way.

So releasing tension releases energy?

Yes, it does. The energy we store as tension becomes available for other uses, such as increasing our awareness and perception. Let's leave that until later, though. For now, let's focus on releasing tension and making space in the body.

Making space?

If tension is contraction, then releasing tension is expansion. The spine is a set of rings held tightly together. When we begin to release the tension holding the rings together we get more space between them. It's very useful to think of working with the body this way: making space in it.

Won't we become formless blobs on the floor if we do that?

Hah! No, not at all. We just aren't wired that way. If anything, we are wired a little too tightly and need to loosen things up!

So how do we start?

You can start anywhere, but there are a few good ways to release lines of tension in the body that pretty much work for everyone.

Begin by lying on your side in the position shown below. When you get stretched out, you'll find the tension raises your head a little.

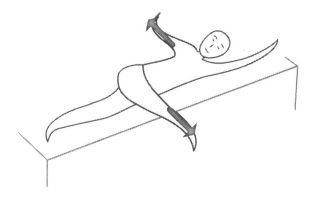

The position of the legs and arms and whether your knees are bent or not is unimportant. Find a position where the tension is more or less evenly distributed from your foot to your head. It should be a position that has tension but is not painful.

When you are stretched out, you will find a line of tension that runs along the top of the upper leg from the foot to the hip, curls underneath your body at the waist and crosses up and over your chest, shoulder and arm.

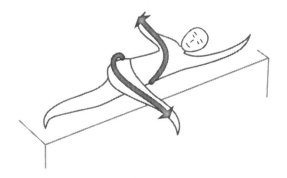

Breathe in, and breathe down through your pelvis towards your feet. (Remember breathing down?)

It may take a couple breaths, but when you breathe down, it becomes possible to stretch the entire line. Your head will drop and your pelvis will move away from your rib cage. Your spine may sway a bit up to your head; let your body move as it wants to. Presto! Instant space between your hips and ribs.

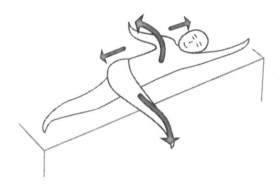

Play with the position a bit, stretch a little more, find a little more tension and breathe down. Feels good, doesn't it?

Try the other side, too!

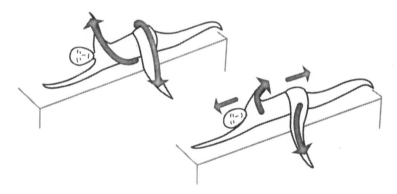

A variation that beautifully works the front line of the body is to arc the upper side of the body and then release. As with the twist, the exact position is not important, simply find the tension in your own body in any position that feels right. The point of your hip will be at the top of the arc.

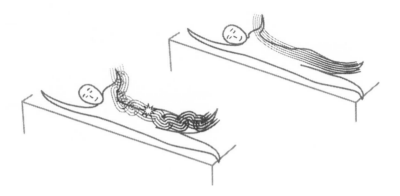

Breathe in and breathe down. Let your body move from the hip. Repeat on the other side!

This works for everybody?

Maybe, maybe not. Every human body on the planet is unique, with a unique set of patterns of tension and energy. What will be a position of tension for one person may not be tense for someone else.

The important thing to remember is that it is YOUR body, and you are seeking to release tension and make space. What you will find is that there is no end to the possible positions! Have fun!

4 Stretch out your pattern

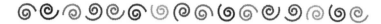

Do we ever really pay much attention to how we sit, stand, and move through our day? When you sit and cross your legs, do you almost always cross the same leg? Do you brush your teeth the same way nine times out of ten?

These are patterns of movement, learned and added on to during our lives. That's why adolescents can seem awkward, where adults move more smoothly: the adults have had more time to refine the patterns of movement in their adult body.

As we learn to move our bodies in certain ways, the body tries to accommodate us. Every night, the body refreshes itself, repairing everything it can. And not only repairing, but growing itself to accommodate what we ask of it.

How much can we ask?

If we ask our muscles to grow bigger and stronger through repetitive work or exercise, that is exactly what the body will try to do. There are limits, of course, because we all have genetic body types that give us our form. If not, short people could grow taller by stretching!

Our bodies adapt as best they can to whatever we ask. If we ask, through day after day of hard labor, for our bodies to carry heavy loads, the muscles along the spine will grow larger and tighten to provide more support. Very good for supporting heavy loads, but causing great lower back problems in later life!

If, instead of carrying heavy loads, we focus all our energy forward, as do so many people in this age of desks and computers, the muscles and fascia rearrange themselves to be able to more comfortably hold a hunched-forward position.

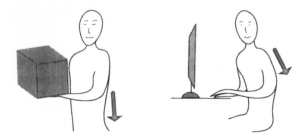

But that's not movement, it's posture...

Exactly! Posture is the locking in of repeated patterns of movement. Have you ever watched a small child walking with a parent? It's endearing to see how the child mimics the gait and body position of the parent, but it is also a glimpse of patterns that become embedded in the child's body, that *become* the child's body as it grows.

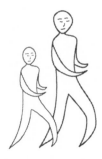

This behavior is probably an ancient survival mechanism of our species. After all, the more the child looks like the adult, the more the adult accepts the child as his/her own. Doesn't every family joke about a child that doesn't fit in as being a changeling?

So the child mimics the parent to fit in.

The child does more than just mimic the parent, the child interacts with every stimulus that shows up. The child reaches out, encounters objects and new information, and reacts accordingly. If the stimulus is pleasurable, the child seeks more of it. If the stimulus is unpleasant, the child seeks to control it, avoid it, or in extreme cases, survive it. The child is constantly growing, creating patterns of interaction, patterns of movement, which solidify into posture and personality.

Think of a child as a young seedling. The instructions for how to grow are already in the plant, but how the plant actually grows depends on so many things: how much sunshine, how much rain, the minerals in the soil, whether anything nibbles on it or steps on it. There is no argument between nature and nurture: it's a multidimensional conversation!

I never thought of myself as a plant!

The process of evolving through time is similar for everything. Even rocks buried deep in the earth feel the tug of earth's gravity, the sun's gravity, the motion of the planet, magnetic fields, and cosmic radiation passing through it from the rest of the universe.

So now I'm like a rock?

In more ways than you might think! But let's return to the child. A child is more complex than a plant, because it grows

in a human environment with lots of cross-currents. If you
grow up with a fearful parent who is always on edge, how
can you not tune to that vibration? You will learn to jump at
sounds, and your body will grow itself to be able to jump away
from danger, even if the jumping you do is inward rather than
physical.

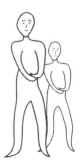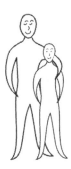

If you grow up in a loving family, will you not be more
open to sharing love? Your body will be more open to the
world, the chest wider, the shoulders straighter and more
relaxed, your stance more solid.

We are what happens to us, then.

Many have said that, and we all know people who attribute
their current life to everything that has happened to them.
   We are not, however, tablets of wax that take impressions,
we are growing patterns of energy with self- awareness. A
plant that is stepped on hard will be twisted out of true, but
it will continue to grow, and its own internal instructions will
try to straighten things out. Humans are much more complex;
we twist and straighten our channels and structures to find the
best accommodation with the world in which we live.
   No one lives in exactly the same world, not even identical
twins, so every single human pattern is unique. Every pattern

has its own twists and turns; like the unfolding of a flower, we unfold into time, each in our own way.

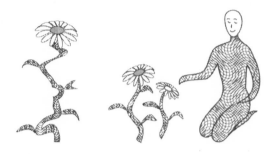

You said we twist and straighten our own channels...

Yes. A child denied love may spend his/her life seeking love. With severe trauma, the child may close their patterns up, reject all interaction, and spend their life gazing at their hurt places.

Others will twist their patterns less tightly. They might manipulate people to give them attention without having to give anything in return. Still others will focus their patterns to project love in order to get others to give it back to them.

Many people find outside patterns that help straighten out their channels. It might be religion, psychotherapy, adopted/extended family, meditation, yoga or any number of things that work out the kinks from past hurt and trauma. Straightening the channels re-directs the energy in us so that it flows more easily.

How does it work?

Everything is connected in the body: all the energy centers of base, sex, breath, heart, speech, mind, and crown. We can try to straighten our channels with methods that focus on one center. Many people do, trying to re-wire themselves through their thoughts, or through meditating on the universe, or opening their heart.

These are all good! They all work, but it is harder to straighten out a blanket by grabbing one corner and shaking it than it is to shake it by two corners.

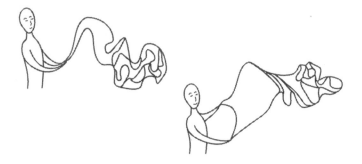

And the easiest and most effective of all is to grab all four corners and pull all of them at the same time.

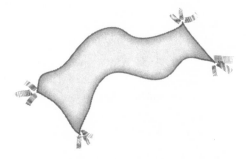

So in Tantra, we grab as many corners as we can, shaking and straightening the blanket side to side, corner to corner. Let's start with the neck and shoulders, and the geometry of tension.

5 The geometry of tension

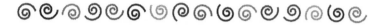

When we feel a pain in the body, we usually feel it as a point. It may be very large point, but it seems separate from the rest of the body, as if it is a separate place. We often experience our bodies this way even when we are not in pain.

Try it for yourself. Hold your arm out and feel through your palm, as if you are touching air. There is a huge number of muscles and bones involved, but what you are feeling is your palm!

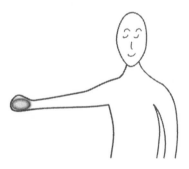

This is one-dimensional tension, the sensation of feeling a point in your body. This is default mode for many people.

Default mode?

Yes. Many people experience their bodies as a succession of points, their awareness moving from one point to the next. We can also experience, and keep track of, much more than one point.

How?

Simply settle yourself comfortably so that you are steady and balanced. Extend your arm again and feel your palm. While holding the feeling in your palm, feel your head. You now have two points in your body you are tracking. Connect the points and let yourself feel your whole arm from head to palm.

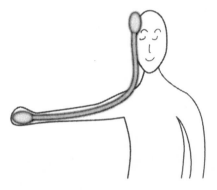

The moment you shift your awareness to the whole arm, it will drop and relax slightly. That's because the muscles concerned with holding the whole arm are subtly different than the muscles concerned with feeling the palm.

You've just woken up part of your body! Try it again, for once is interesting, but twice means it's real and that you can find it again.

You can feel multiple lines, too. A good example is the head, neck and shoulders. We all carry tension there.

Tilt your head to one side and stretch out the opposite shoulder. Stretch until you feel some tension.

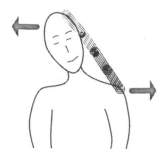

Feel the line of tension between the tip of your shoulder and side of your head. This line will feel like a taut bowstring holding the bow of your head, neck and shoulders.

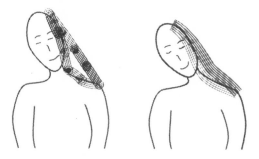

Good! Now breathe in, and breathe down, letting the bowstring relax.

You may need to work at it a bit, but when you get it there is an unmistakable sensation of making space between your shoulder and head.

Try it a couple times to make sure you have it. It's now only fair to do the other side!

What just happened?

The energy in your body exists in not just points, not just lines, but in more complex structures as well. And as we have just seen, part of the structure can even be outside the physical skin!

It's very hard to relax a single point, but much easier to relax lines and structures. The larger and more complex the structure, the more energy it has, and the greater release you can get. That's much of the reason that yogis get into such complicated positions, because there is much more energy available. It can be enough to launch you into the universe.

Do I have to become a yogi, then?

Hah! No, not at all, though it a fine thing to be. The point is to be conscious, the position you use to get there is actually irrelevant. In fact, yogis often approach this from the other direction: the physical demands they place upon their bodies open up a lot of energy, which hopefully punches open their consciousness. Much better to work directly on being conscious!

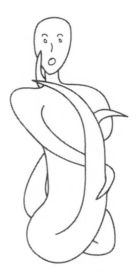

How does releasing energy increase your consciousness?

It doesn't, not by itself. It is just that much of our energy, and a lot of our awareness, is taken up with maintaining the tension in our bodies. If we reduce the tension, we have more energy and more awareness available.

In a way, you could say that releasing locked-up energy increases our awareness because we have more information.

More information?

Some scientists have speculated, and some have flatly pronounced, that energy is information. To understand how, we have to back up a step.

Quantum mechanics has long known that the way we look at something determines what we see. The same phenomenon can be seen as either a particle or a wave. It is neither: the form it takes and how you work with it depends on how you view it.

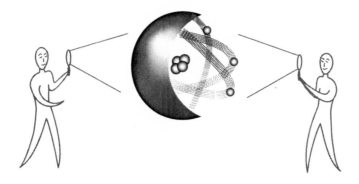

That makes sense because we know that what we call matter is also what we call energy. Einstein explained it in

1905, and forty years later humans proved it in the atom bomb.

Energy and information have the same relationship as energy and matter. Look at an energy flow from one direction and it is energy. Another way, it is information.

It may seem a strange concept, yet we use it all the time. A star that radiates energy into a telescope is read as information about the star. The look we send to a friend is read perfectly. The pain energy we feel is a cry for attention.

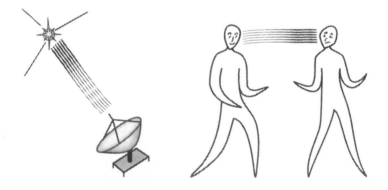

Matter, energy, information. Each perspective is useful. The muscles release, the energy releases, information releases.

For now, let's turn back to the physical level, back to geometry and the triangle.

6 Triangulate

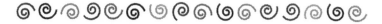

Triangles are as easy to work with as our bow and bowstring. An easy triangle to work with is the one formed when you hold your foot out with your hand. You don't need your leg straight, you simply need tension on the leg and arm.

Sit comfortably cross-legged on a bed or the floor. Or a pillow. Or sit in a chair! Breathe in, and breathe down.

Grab hold of your foot (the big toe is good to hold onto!). Look at the triangle formed by the position. One side is your leg, one side is your arm, and the third side is your side. Don't worry if any of them are bent or curved, just feel for the lines of tension in the triangle.

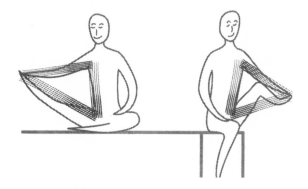

Stretch the triangle a bit, distributing the tension evenly. You may be able to wave the triangle around a bit, but it will feel awkward, because it is still anchored by the pelvis.

Breathe in, and breathe down through your pelvis. Your sit
bones will drop, and the triangle will begin to flex and move.
Watch what it does!

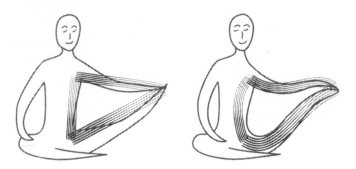

Play with it, feel how your arm and leg move. Feel how the
tension on your spine changes with the movement. When you
are ready, stretch out a little to increase the tension on your
spine. This creates a bigger triangle with your spine as one
side. Breathe in and breathe down, and let your spine go.

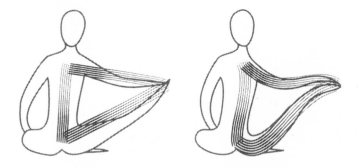

Pretty cool, huh? You can't help but bend and wave in a
way you probably haven't done since you were a little child.
And that means that this movement is a pattern you haven't
touched in a very long time. You could call it "straightening
out your patterns."

The patterns from childhood?

Maybe, or from any where/time in your life. We have to start from wherever it is we are now, which usually means working backwards towards our childhood, sorting through persistent patterns. Sometimes, if we have a strong childhood or adolescent pattern in us, we might discover a great deal of tension very quickly!

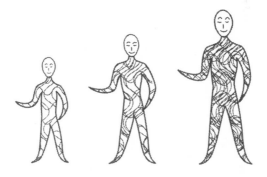

What happens then?

Well, the first thing that happens is that we release a lot of energy that has been tied up for a long time. The initial release can be euphoric. It's very possible that some of the energy generated by the physical release is in the form of internal chemicals like endorphins that make us feel good. That is, incidentally, why many athletes get addicted to physical activity: a good shot of endorphins is a real high, and a great antidote to modern stress.

It is much better to release tension consciously. In order to connect to the universe, we need to straighten out our energy patterns, not overlay repetitive endorphin production on top of them as a feel-good escape!

But isn't euphoria good?

Euphoria is a lovely state! But you can't live in the universe in only one state; there's too much energy and change in the universe for that. If the universe is changing states constantly, so must we who live in it, if we are to live richly and well-tuned.

Well-tuned?

Well-tuned. But let's save that for another time and go back to that initial release of energy. When we release tension, it feels great. Our whole body moves into a calmer state, maybe with a slight high from endorphins. The spine relaxes, feels more flexible, moves more easily. If we open our eyes widely, we can expand our senses and feel larger.

Can't stay there, though. Wish we could, because it is a really nice place to hang out! At the moment we recognize that we feel great, the mind kicks in and starts talking to us.

Go away! But the moment is gone. That's okay, though, because we can return whenever we want to.

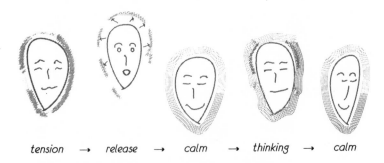

tension → release → calm → thinking → calm

Indeed, life seems to be a process of switching states, of switching channels back and forth from the body to bliss to the mind and on to whatever is next. That's called unfolding in time.

Unfolding in time...

A fancy way of saying that everything is always changing, but with the understanding that the unfolding is like the growth of a plant, pushing upward and outward.

It's okay to go back into your mind. That's where most of us live most of the time and it's a great place. It's just not the only place we're allowed to live.

If you push the limits with drugs or forced exercises to feel larger, you can increase the chances of a rubber band recoil. The harder you push out, the harder is the rebound back into the mind.

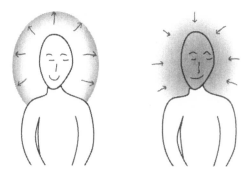

This rubber band effect can actually limit our perception to two end-states.

Love/hate is a good example. Who doesn't know a child who loves something one day and hates it the next? We all know people who get stuck in one channel, until something jars them and they flip the switch to something else. A lot of people bounce back and forth without really knowing they are doing so!

It makes more sense to move purposefully from state to state. Stretch and release the energy, enjoy the feeling, bounce back into the moment, stretch again, or not...

Speaking of stretching, we have one happy leg and one jealous leg, so treat your other side with the same exquisite attention you just gave to the first side!

And see what else you can find in the exploring...

7 Finding your truth:
Socrates meets Shakti

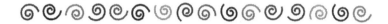

Tantra is more of an attitude or an orientation than it is a system, tradition or methods. When we say that there are no rules in Tantra, we really mean it! But what is it we mean?

Rules are boundaries that define what we should and shouldn't do. They are like the lines on a highway that keep us driving in one direction in straight lines.

No one would argue that lines on a highway are not necessary and good things, or that we should ignore them. If a rule is practical, and works, we should use it to navigate the world. But rules can also keep us traveling the same pathways over and over again, until the way is so ingrained that we don't think about it any more.

And many of the rules we create are not just dotted lines on a highway, but walls that block our vision and make us go one way or another without us realizing it. Imagine being lost in a maze of alleyways, or in the middle of a room full of office cubicles. From inside, you can't see the way out, but if you rise out of the maze and see it from above, the path would be perfectly clear.

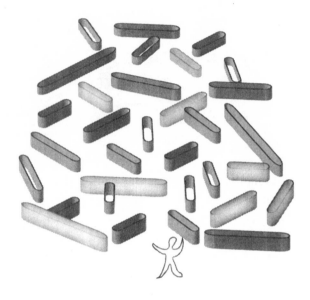

So we have to rise above our mazes?

Yes! The mazes we encounter everyday in our own behavior are composed of rules we have made or adopted. If you can't see the pattern of the rules you've adopted, you're going to spend a lot of time walking into the walls of your own rules.

What happens then?

You might get pulled up short so you turn away in a different direction. You might break your own rules, punching a hole in the energy of that pattern in your body. If you punch through it often enough, it becomes a mere outline that you think you still believe in.

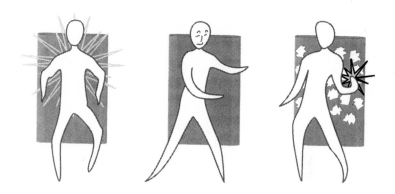

Is Tantra, then about breaking the rules?

That's a very good question. For some people that might actually be true. For example, they might have a set of rules in their head about sex. They might use Tantra as a way to break the rules. Breaking rules is excellent if it leads to liberation, but not so good if you are just massaging (and reinforcing) patterns mixing guilt and pleasure.

How can you tell the difference?

Ah, this is where Socrates meets Shakti! Socrates was an ancient Greek philosopher who carried on dialogues with his students, questioning their assumptions relentlessly. This method of inquiry became known in the Western world as the Socratic Dialogue. Socrates was very popular with his students, but the elected authorities made him drink poison to get rid of him.

Shakti is the feminine principle of Tantra. The ancient texts say that Shiva, the god of creation, created Shakti from a bone in his body in order to have a conversation. The conversation that has come down to us is considered to be a guide to enlightenment.

It makes one wonder if the story of Shiva/Shakti was re-written by men long after the oral tradition started. Given the paramount importance of women yoginis in the early tradition, it seems much more likely that Shakti created Shiva, rather than the other way around!

This is Socratic: to question what you have been told, and seek to discover the truth for yourself.

So you discover for yourself whether you are liberating yourself or just breaking the rules?

Exactly.

How?

By checking in with yourself and asking if you are really feeling what you think you are feeling, and why.

Give me an example.

Say something.

Okay. I feel great!

Good. Why do you feel great?

I just do!

What do you feel when you are not feeling great?

Uh.... Not so great.

What does that feel like?

Maybe low on energy, maybe feeling like things are not going my way.

What kinds of things don't go your way?

Relationships, my job, having enough money, and my drawing isn't as good.

Would you say that relationships, job, money and drawing are "your way?"

Well it's more than just those things... it's everything.

So if everything is not "going your way," it might mean that things are bypassing you, going around you; that you feel disconnected a little from everything.

Yes. Exactly.

And feeling great is when you feel that you are connected to everything...

Yes.

There really aren't any other questions to ask. This is as far as the Socratic method can take us. We have taken what appeared to be an absolute statement, explored what we really meant by it, and arrived at the point where we must turn to the universe for answers. We are now in the realm of the Shakti, in the realm of connecting to the universe.

We ask the universe for the answer?

We can! And very often the universe will answer, if not directly, than through the words of another person, or an event that causes change in our lives.

If we ask the universe for things that the universe agrees with, we often get them. If we ask for things that are not in accord with the Goddess's intent, we encounter things very much un-looked for! It often seems to be the case that we do not get what we ask for, but instead something else that we didn't know we actually needed more!

So the universe answers...

This seems like a strange notion, and yet we all believe it. William James, one of the founders of Pragmatism, said that truth is what works in the long run. What has had a longer run than the idea that the universe talks to us? Spirits, sprites, shamans, trees, gods and goddesses, the void, mathematics: if it is so deeply embedded in human culture that the universe talks to us, maybe we should give it a go and see what happens!

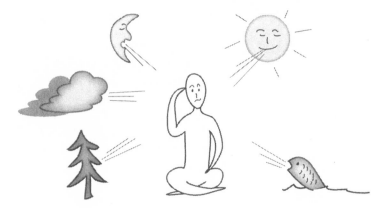

You're not serious...

Actually, I am. But not necessarily in the way you might think. The Goddess is not in the business of answering all our questions; she is, after all, busy running and expanding the whole universe. Directing traffic, if you will!

Humans are in the universe, we are of it. We already have a huge number of answers; *we have more rules in all our traditions than we know what to do with.*

What do you mean?

Humans have filled many libraries with rules for living. All religions have them, all traditions have them, most philosophies have them. Families have them, communities have them, schools have them, businesses have them, governments have them. We are drowning in rules for living.

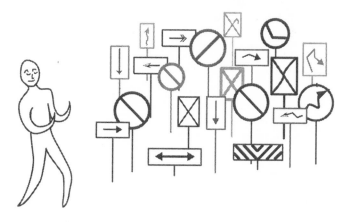

There is a story of a young child entering a room full of horse manure. The child cries out in happiness. When asked why, the reply was "With all this horse manure, there must be a pony in here somewhere!"

Like the child, we are convinced that somewhere in all
the rules is an answer. When, in fact, any answers we need are
already in us, and in the universe.

So how do we find them?

By sorting through what we are really feeling and thinking.
Not accepting assertions, but questioning if what we think we
feel is really what we feel.

It is very easy, to feel a thing and accept it without
questioning. Many people will declare they are hurt by
someone else's actions. Consider how an internal questioning
might go:

I feel hurt!

Why?

That person was rude to me!

Why does that hurt?

Everyone feels free to dump on me. I don't like it!

Have a lot of people dumped on me?

Yes. Well, not everybody, but a lot of people.

Well, why do they do it?

They probably don't mean to, but they're not being nice!

Why should they be nice?

Because I deserve it!

Aha! Why do I deserve it?

Because I think I deserve more from the universe than I
get.

Now we're getting somewhere.

Now we are getting to the original pattern of this feeling, a pattern that has come from our childhood experiences, or adolescent experiences, or handed to us by some tradition that we have accepted.

If you think about it, this kind of feeling could not be from the universe itself. If the universe is the only game in town, why would we think we deserve more? Do we think we know better how to manage things? Not very likely, is it?

But this basic feeling is sitting there like a lump in my throat...

Remember when we talked about grabbing all the corners of a blanket and shaking and smoothing it out? Well, asking questions and probing your own feelings and thoughts is only one corner of the blanket.

Another corner of the blanket is breathing down and letting your energy connect to the ground the universe created for us.

Grab another corner by stretching out the pattern of this feeling. If you're feeling strong emotions, or running around in your mind like a rat in a maze, you are activating an energy pattern in your body. You have to be, because energy powers everything we do.

Patterns stretch through the whole body, especially the spine and pelvis. If we can feel for the whole pattern of tension in our body, we can stretch it out, remove some of the tension from our childhood, and take another, clearer, look at everything.

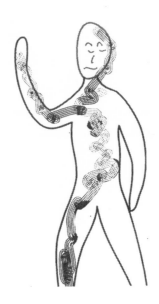

Let's do it!

Bring to mind something that is troubling you, something about which you have strong feelings, be it family, friends, work, or something that happened just today.

Stretch out your body and look for a position that seems to correspond to the tension your thoughts or emotions have produced. It might be a front line, a back line, or a line that twists around you a bit.

Stretch to increase the tension, feeling for one endpoint of the pattern in your head: there will be one part of your head that feels tenser than the rest. Look for the other endpoint. If you've got the pattern stretched out, you will feel tension all the way to your pelvis or even your feet.

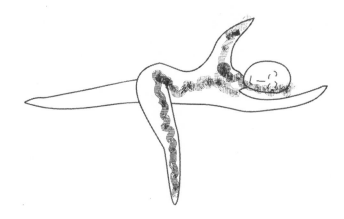

When you find a line of tension that seems to connect to your feeling, breathe in, and breathe down, releasing the pattern and releasing the tension in your body.

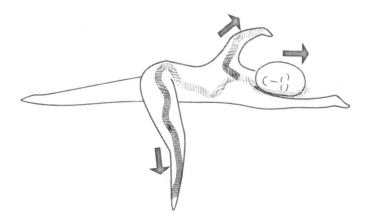

You are tugging on your mind with your body, and your body with your mind. Much more effective than dealing with only one at a time!

This is using our awareness and mind to identify the real source of the tension, and then using the energy of the universe, the Shakti, in your own body to release the tension. You will be surprised at the answers you find! Not to mention the increased clarity and calm.

So that's the answer from the universe?

To get an answer you have to ask the right question. We now know that we have lots of rules that inhibit our clear seeing and moving. That we can ask questions of ourselves to identify what we are really feeling. That we can straighten out the pattern by straightening out the energy in it.

Once we get some clarity and calm, we can begin to recognize much more clearly the answers we get from the universe. And we'll find that the universe talks to us in many, many ways.

8 The body as wiring

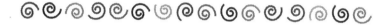

When we stop and ask questions of ourselves to figure out what we are really thinking or feeling, it seems easy to ask questions and work our way down to bedrock. Why is it we don't think this way all the time?

Mind is a complicated place. Our minds run away with us, we are out of our minds when we are crazy, we are of two minds when we can't make a decision, and we have a meeting of the minds when we agree on something. Our minds certainly seem to be very busy all of the time!

Integrating mind and body is very hard to do in the mind. Let's look instead at the mind IN the body.

To begin with, we have three brains. They are commonly referred to as the reptile, mammal and human brains. In anatomy, they roughly correspond to the medulla oblongata, cerebellum, and cerebrum. We can think of the human brain as a enhanced primate version, with lots more processing power and new functions.

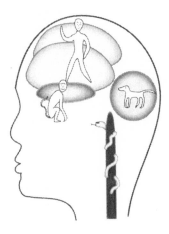

The reptilian brain is, you guessed it, the eldest. It is similar in structure to the brains of reptiles and is directly descended from our reptilian ancestors.

Reptilian ancestors?

Of course! Life on earth started as single-cell organisms in the sea, and evolved through sea creatures, amphibians, reptiles, and mammals. The history of where our species has been is written not only in the geologic record, but also in our DNA and the structures and functions of our body.

Why?

Evolution is what works, what survives. Each structure in our body is the result of experimentation over 3.5 billion years of life. What has survived is what worked over the long run. It is not an accident that humans are the most successful species on the planet, colonizing almost every micro-climate and finding enough energy not only to feed ourselves but to support civilizations.

We have been successful because we incorporated what works. One of those things is a reptile brain!

It gives us most of our basic functions, like breathing, really fast emergency responses that by-pass the other brains, and the main wiring of our bodies, which is the spinal cord of movement and information.

Aren't reptiles vicious?

Reptiles are never vicious, but they play to survive! Don't blame anger and cruelty on the reptile brain because it isn't wired for those kinds of emotions. The reptile brain gives you the ability to do certain things. What you do with it, what kind of energy you run through it, is up to you.

And the mammal brain?

The cerebellum helps coordinate movement and a number of warm-blooded functions. The cerebellum exists in amphibians and reptiles, but evolved to encompass memory and recognition by the time mammals appeared. And patterns such as family, herd, and pack behavior.

The primate part of the human brain provides the circuits for primate behavior that seem to be hard-wired into humans: curiosity, family, extended family, tribal patterns. Patterns of aggression and display, grooming behavior, mating behavior.

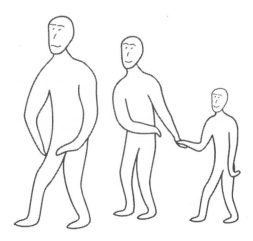

We're hard-wired for behaviors?

Oh yes, these are basic human patterns you see in every single culture humans have ever created. If it is everywhere, it has to in some fashion be embedded in our wiring.

And the human brain?

Ah! The human brain is the big processor, with room for lots of thoughts and patterns, and an extraordinary ability to connect the rest of the wiring.

What exactly is wiring?

Wiring is a very useful word that helps remind us of several things. The first is that energy runs in patterns in our bodies, much like electricity runs through the wires in a building.

The second is that wires carry both information and energy. In a computer, circuits carry electrical impulses that can be decoded as information. So too does the wiring in our bodies. In fact the model for the most advanced new networks of computers are *neural nets* patterned after the neural networks in our brains.

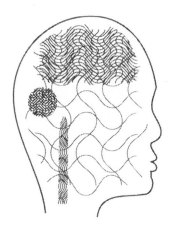 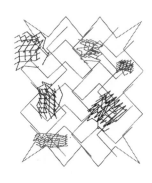

Wiring is usually rated for a certain amount of energy. If there is too much energy, you can burn out your wiring. To handle more energy, you will need to upgrade your wiring. If you want to change the pattern of the electricity, you may need to re-wire your circuits.

In the body, there is the physical wiring that we can map as nerves which pass electricity from living cell to living cell. Deeper yet, there is the pattern of electrical charges of every atom connected to other atoms.

Yes, wiring is a good term for our modern understanding of the body!

On a practical level...

On a practical level, we have already learned how to release energy in our bodies, running it down to connect to the ground, and letting it run up our spines to our heads. We have begun to re-wire circuits in our bodies by finding lines of tension, stretching them out, and releasing them. We have held our bodies in new positions, created new patterns of movement, and created new pathways and connections.

The real connection between mind and body is electric!

Mind and body? How?

We've already seen how thoughts and emotions are part of patterns in the body that we can explore and release, like straightening out our blanket. But we can also use the mind and body directly with each other by folding the blanket and connecting two places.

Let's try a simple demonstration. Let's introduce our head to our knee. Don't laugh! At least not until you've tried it.

Okay.

Settle yourself cross-legged or in a chair. Prop your knee up if that is more comfortable for you.

Breathe in, and breathe down.

Lean to one side, head towards knee. Breathe in, and breathe down, lowering your head to your knee. It may take a couple breaths to get there. Since the exact position isn't important, feel free to use a block or pillow, or just bring your knee up to your head.

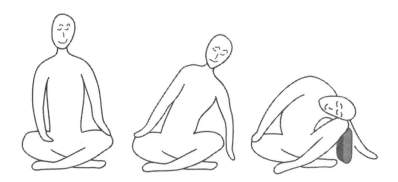

Move your head around and feel your knee. What does the knee feel like? Can you feel the skin sliding over the kneecap?

Breathe in and breathe down, switching your awareness to your knee. Use your knee to feel your head, moving the knee against your cheekbone or jaw or brow. Breathe in and breathe down, leaving your head and knee together.

Move your awareness back to your head (something we are all good at!), breathe in and breathe out from your head towards your knee. Keep going until the knee feels held and cradled by your head and your head feels much bigger than it usually does!

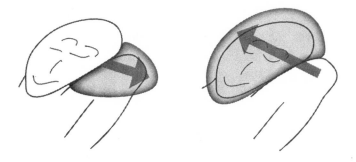

Switch your awareness back to your knee. Breathe in, and breathe out from your knee into your head, and keep going until it feels like your head is being held and cradled by your knee.

Breathe in, and breathe down, relaxing both head and knee. Gently let the two boundaries become one boundary around both head and knee.

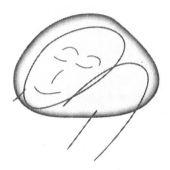

An indescribable feeling, isn't it? We've probably put our head and knee together many times in our life, but never since early childhood with the deliberate intent of exploring what it feels like, and what they feel like joined together.

This is literally connecting the mind and the body!

You can do this with hand to foot, ankle to knee, elbow to thigh. Although you are not literally using your head, your mind helps visualize the connection.

This connection, this joining, is aware exploration, and an excellent jumping off point for everything else we will explore.

So go introduce your head to your other knee. And to the rest of your body. Here's a hint: there doesn't have to be a physical connection...

9 The latest download...

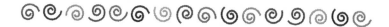

All the things we've done so far... do you do them every day?

Yes. Every day. More than once a day. Breathe in and breathe down. Find lines of tension and release them. Find patterns and release them. Find thoughts and emotions, relate them to the body, and release them.

To re-wire the patterns?

You can think of it that way, though it might be more accurate to say that constant exploration just keeps growing your patterns. Most of us tend to do similar things every day and deal with similar issues. Every-day similarities beat a path through us.

Explore in different ways, and there is no end to the ways you can explore your mind and body.

Sounds like a lot of work...

More like play! Or work and play together. Or just exploring, like we did as young children when every movement, every pattern, was new.

Want to reclaim your childhood? Reclaim with awareness the movements you made all those years ago!

By all means take as much time exploring as you can, but you can wring out the day in a few minutes. A few minutes breathing in and breathing down, a few spine twists and stretches, and the day's patterns will fall away, leaving you more relaxed, lighter, and clearer.

That's nice, but where is this getting us?

In a word, to the universe. But to understand why and how, we have to talk about what science has discovered in the last few decades.

Since the dawn of human civilization, humans have tried to understand how it is they exist in the world, and what it means. We have created so many stories, so many beautiful myths and images to explain it all. Most of it was based on some kind of empirical evidence, some people journeying out into the universe to bring back a new image, a new pattern.

With the development of science and scientific methods, we found a way to begin testing our assumptions about the world, rather than relying on the insights of a few great teachers and mystics.

Teachers and mystics had empirical evidence?

They had their own radical experiences with the universe. The word radical means "of the root." They went back to the source and brought back new insights.

How is science different?

Science explicitly declares its assumptions, creates a hypothesis, and then sets out to test it, either through physical experiments or through mathematics. Over time, the hypotheses become more and more accurate, because science discards explanations that do not work. What we have at any given moment is our best guess at how the universe really works. And the latest download from the universe is quite revolutionary...

Latest download?

Well, we have to back up a bit to make sense of it. After Albert Einstein defined his famous equation $E=mc^2$, which described the relationship of matter and energy, he turned his attention to the cosmos.

Einstein created equations that described the movement of the universe. Everyone knows about the Big Bang, which proposes that the universe exploded from a single point, and is now exploding out in all directions. Einstein sought to describe that movement through the interaction of many variables, among them the amount of matter in the universe.

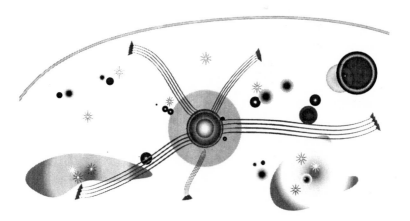

Einstein's cosmological theories were both right and wrong, and drove physicists crazy for decades. The problem, you see, was that all the variations of the theory assumed the universe contained more matter than anybody could actually find!

So scientists measured and measured and measured, and argued quite a bit, as well. In 2006, a group of scientists announced that they had finally found the missing matter.

They called it *dark energy*, and it is stitched into all space/time, not only the spaces between the stars, but also the spaces inside the atoms of our bodies. Physicists have called it the *fabric of the universe*.

While visible matter comprises just 4% of the universe, a form of dark energy called dark matter comprises 23%, and dark energy makes up the rest.

Dark energy is indeed the fabric of the universe if it makes up 96% of everything!

Dark energy is scientifically proven?

The scientists think so! The reason it is called dark energy is because we can't actually see it. To be more accurate, we have not quite yet devised instruments capable of measuring it, although we can infer the existence of dark energy from measuring cosmic background radiation from the Big Bang. You might wonder, then, if it is proven at all. It is. It exists, because if it didn't exist, the universe could not move as it does. Sometimes, this is as close as science can get.

Don't take my word for it, search it up on the internet!

So there is dark energy everywhere.

Everywhere. If everything is made of atoms, then what are atoms made of? They are mostly space, with some protons and neutrons in the middle, and electrons flying around in orbits. But they are mostly space, and space is not a void, but filled with dark energy. There is nothing we can think of that is not made up mostly of space and of dark energy. And that means that there is nothing that is not connected. Let's re-phrase that: everything is connected.

Connected by dark energy.

Dark energy is the most widespread form of energy in the universe, so we might as well just call it the energy of the universe.

Think of it, the energy coursing through your body is the same as the energy holding together the chair you are sitting on, the table in front of you, this book you are reading.

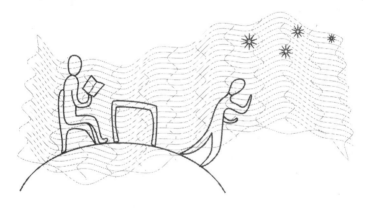

The energy in you is the same energy as in the stars, the same energy as in the earth, the same energy as in that mean man who lives down the street. Turns out all those religions were right: God is everywhere.

Whoa... how did we get from energy to God?

Culture. We talked at the beginning about how our experience of the universe does not take place in a vacuum. Actually, now we know it takes place in a sea of energy!

Culture influences our choice of words and images, even when we are in the midst of changing the culture. All of the spiritual traditions of humans have assumed that everything in the universe is somehow connected. We now have a word for it: energy. What is revolutionary is that we KNOW it exists, it has to exist, and while we can and have denied the existence of God, there is no doubt that the universe is connected by energy.

Fine, everything is connected by energy. How does that change things?

Well, it actually doesn't change anything at all. The universe is still the universe. But we can think about it differently now.

The classic scientific view of the universe is often called "Newtonian" after the great scientist Sir Isaac Newton. The Newtonian universe was like a giant billiard table, where galaxies bounce off each other like billiard balls, and in-between there is only the void of space. There was a fixed, objective set of rules by which it ran, much like a clock.

Now we know that we are not living in a mechanistic Newtonian universe with a set of fixed rules. Now we know that we are living in a sea of energy, and we are not separate from that energy.

What could this mean to us?

We watch the waves of the ocean, and understand that in most waves, the water is not moving at all. Instead, energy is moving through the water molecules, lifting them up and down in a cyclical motion. The water molecules stay where they are, the energy rolls through.

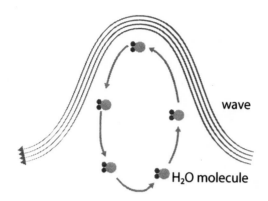

wave

H_2O molecule

We are, if you will, like those waves. We are a standing wave pattern of energy, of information. The pattern is powered by the energy in the sea, but remains in a (reasonably) stable configuration.

A standing wave pattern...

Yes. A wave pattern that looks like a human, is human. Powered by the universe. A universe that is within us as well as outside us. All we have to do is connect the two with our awareness.

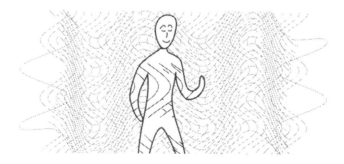

Note on Science:

Current theories in physics of the expanding universe
and the role played by dark energy have moved far beyond
Einstein's original conception. Physicists suspect that the
forces we understand today may be reflections of an even
more fundamental unity in the universe.

10 Tuning your awareness

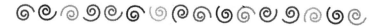

What is awareness? The dictionaries circle around words such as mindfulness, consciousness, wakefulness, and attention, like signs pointing to a scenic spot. We know what all these words refer to because we have been there, we have *experienced* this state.

We are all aware, and experience moments of greater awareness, when patterns fall into place and we think or feel something new and different, or notice something as if for the first time.

What is it we can be aware of? A falling leaf in autumn, how the sunlight sparkles on a pool of water, a quality to someone we had not previously noticed, a pattern of behavior we recognize because we have seen it before. All of these are a focusing of body and mind.

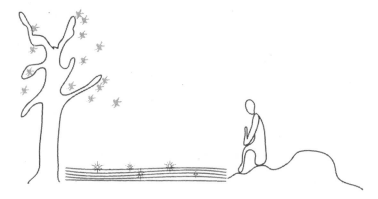

We focus on things constantly, naturally.

Much of the time, we focus with a hum already in our heads, a hum produced by what we wanted to do yesterday and didn't, by what we want that we don't have, by what we want to do next. That hum is our pattern of this moment, constantly changing, and constantly dispersing our focus.

Dispersing?

Dispersed in the sense that we are trying to focus on something while we are thinking and feeling many other things. How many times have you talked to someone while:

- Still being irritated by an incident earlier that day?
- Thinking about whether or not you like this person?
- Wondering if they like you?
- Wondering why they don't like you?
- Thinking of what you want to say next?

We could go on, but we already have five things besides the actual conversation!

To be focused in your awareness is just that: tuning your lens so that you are looking at what you want to be looking at. Everyone can train their awareness on a single thing, on multiple things at the same time, or on a whole field of things.

Like focusing a lens on a camera?

Very much so. We are on auto-focus most of the time, where whatever is moving in the picture grabs our attention. Like digital cameras, we can use portrait mode, where we focus solely on a person, with everything else as indistinct background. Or we can use landscape mode, where we focus on the whole scene.

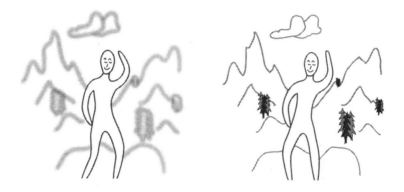

Focusing a lens is a very good description, because our eyes take in frequencies and patterns of light, and focusing a lens allows us to pick and choose which patterns we want to examine.

But we sense frequencies with more than just our eyes. We sense frequencies with all of the energy centers of our bodies. So it might be more accurate and useful to talk about tuning our awareness rather than focusing our awareness.

How do we tune our awareness?

We've already begun! Breathing down, stretching our energy patterns, asking questions. Really, all kinds of ways have been invented. Different traditions use sounds, images, chants. Ceremonies involve a group of people contributing their energy and tuning to the same frequency. Doesn't matter if it is a religious ceremony, a group meditation or chant, or a public singing of the national anthem. The ceremony tunes individuals to the group, creating a more powerful sensing mechanism than most people can create on their own. That's why ceremonies (and riots) are so powerful, and leave us exhilarated.

If you are really going to tune your awareness, though, at some point you have to deal with your own wiring. And that means paying exquisite attention to your energy centers.

What exactly is an energy center?

Simply put, it is a place in the body where a lot of energy lines and patterns cross. The word in Eastern tradition is *chakra*, which is as good a word as any, so we'll use that word a lot, too.

Different systems identify different numbers of chakras, and ascribe different qualities and colors to each. For our purposes, let's stick with the seven well known ones numbered from 1 at the bottom of the spine to 7 at the top of the head. Below are the numbers and the names we'll use.

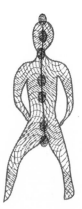

7. crown chakra
6. mind chakra
5. throat chakra

4. heart chakra
3. breath chakra

2. second chakra
1. base chakra

Tuning a chakra is really just bringing your awareness to that chakra and exploring it. Let's start with the two most people know best, the heart and the mind.

Sit comfortably, breathe in and breathe down. Your spine will straighten, your head will move back and up, and you may feel the top of your head relax.

Breathe in, and breathe out through the front of your heart.

We're not, of course, physically breathing out through our heart, but you'll be surprised at how much it feels that way!

Your chest will relax and expand, and your next breath will feel much easier and lighter.

Breathe in and breathe down, savoring the moment.

Breathe in, and now breathe out through the back of your heart. It may take a few breaths, but you should feel the same sense of relaxing and expanding in your back as in your chest. It's very peaceful, isn't it?

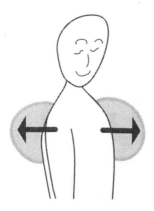

We can do this with each of our energy centers. Let's try the mind next.

Breathe in and breathe down. Breathe in, and breathe out through the front of your head. It may feel forced at first, the muscles of your face may feel tight. As you breathe, just let your face and the front of your head widen a little bit with each breath.

When you are ready, breathe out through the back of your head, taking your time, letting it happen rather than trying to

make it happen. When you have opened the back, your head
will feel like a ring with an empty middle.

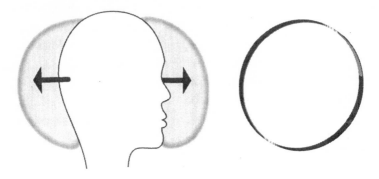

This is tuning your mind to the energy of the universe.
The empty space inside the ring of your head is not empty! It
is filled with the energy that is in everything.

It's a lovely feeling...

Isn't it? The experience is lovely enough to keep millions
of people meditating every day. It's why the Zen tradition
places so much emphasis on clear mind and empty mind. But
even if the mind is one of our most powerful and familiar
energy centers, there are many energy centers, not just one.
And we want to go for broadband!

Broadband, like connecting to the internet?

Yes, although we are concerned not just with download
speeds, but also with bandwidth, the range of frequencies
we can access. Each of the energy centers in our body are
tuned to a different set of frequencies. Rely on any one set of
frequencies for too long, and you begin to limit yourself by
improving some frequencies and letting others fade away.

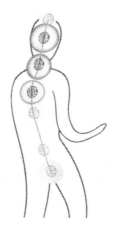

So we move on?

Yes! Let's try the throat chakra.

Breathe in and breathe down, centering yourself.

Breathe in and breathe out through the front of your throat.

Breathe in and breathe out through the back of the throat.

We've now opened three energy centers that lie in a row: the heart, throat and mind. The energy center at the top is called the crown chakra. It is considered by many people to be a main point of entry to the universe. It certainly is an entry, but higher frequency is not necessarily better, not when you can have broadband.

We've already practiced opening the crown chakra by breathing down. Breathing down creates a corresponding upward movement straight out through the top of our head.

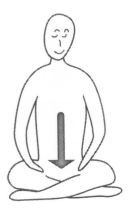
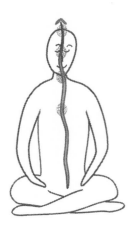

So we'll breathe in and breathe down, paying exquisite attention this time to how the downward movement is followed by an upward movement. With our heart, throat and mind opened, the sensation up from the heart up will be greater. Don't forget to open your heart after you breathe down and the energy starts to rise!

This is an interesting feeling...

It may take some practice to tune your awareness to this sequence, but it indeed feels wonderful. Calm, refreshing, energized, as if you were on another plane. This is a state that is much sought after, consciously in meditative traditions and unconsciously by many others.

Unconsciously sought after?

It feels good, right? It's connecting to some heady frequencies of the universe. All humans are trying to connect to the universe, whether they approach the universe as God, their experience of being cradled by their mother, taking in energy in the form of food or emotion, or the feeling of being caught up in some great endeavor. Each different approach relies on a specific pattern of energy centers.

Some people rely on one energy center. We all know people who spend most of their time in their heart or in their head. We even know people who operate from their throat chakra, and simply never stop talking!

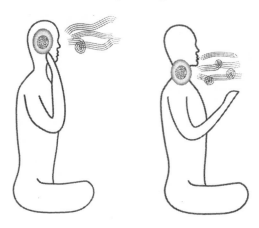

People who spend most of their time in one energy center, one set of frequencies, often find it confusing to deal with any other frequencies.

More commonly, we use a combination of energy centers. A good example is the mind and the throat. That's a combination which is very good for arguing!

Another common combination is the throat and heart, whose combined frequencies are very good for gushing over just about anything.

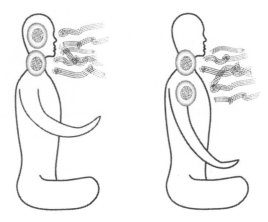

Some people open all four of the upper energy centers. They glow with energy in the upper part of their bodies. They are kind and gentle, but seem a little attenuated, a little pale, as if they are becoming bleached. They float, a little, on the ground, as though their lower bodies are not quite there.

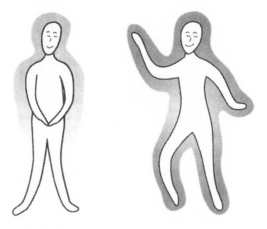

This is connecting to the universe, but with less than broadband. If we've got all these frequencies, why not fire them all up?!

11 Adding your base

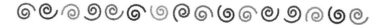

Humans seem to attach much importance to the idea of "higher" and "lower," as if one aspect of the universe could be better than another.

We are wired to perceive duality. We see it everywhere, and it is a very useful tool. We can climb the duality ladder back and forth, grabbing hold of one opposite after another, to the top of whatever we are climbing. This or that. Good or bad. Black or white.

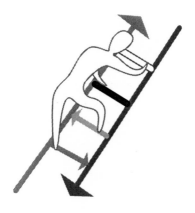

Duality, though, is only two dimensions. And the universe works in more than that. Take black and white. To a human, white is the reflection of all colors and black is the absorption of all colors. But are they opposites? From a human visual point of view they might be. But from an energetic point of view the visual spectrum from human black to human white is only a small part of the whole spectrum of energy.

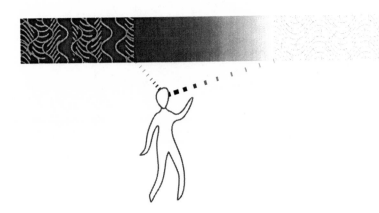

Only black or white? When you are confronted by only two choices, look for another perspective. Rise above the maze to see how the two opposites are related.

Duality is a lot like a hammer. To a hammer, everything is a nail. And you may not be looking at a nail at all...

Sometimes we need a screwdriver?

Sometimes we need a whole tool kit! And we already have one in all the different energy centers, or chakras, in the body. We've worked with opening the chakras from the heart up, let's now explore the three other chakras, starting with the breath. We can locate the breath chakra in the vicinity of the bottom of our sternum, near the diaphragm.

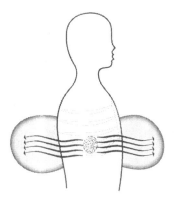

Breathe in and breathe down, centering yourself.

Breathe in and breathe out through the front of your chest below the heart, at the bottom of the sternum. You should feel an opening in the lower ribs, with the shoulders falling back.

Breathe in and breathe down.

Breathe in and breathe out through your back opposite your sternum. Your mid-back should widen, and will probably curl forward as the tension is released.

Breathe in and breathe down.

Now for the second chakra.

The sexual chakra?

So it is often identified, since it provides much of the energy in sex. But that is not the only role it plays, situated as it is in the crossroads, the anchor, of the pelvis.

The second chakra has a powerful effect also because it is often joined with the first chakra. The joining is explicit in many forms of yoga in the mula bandha, the base lock, where you close your base chakra. Instinctively for most humans, the joining happens in the fight-or-flight response, or for sex.

It is so instinctive that many people keep the two chakras close together much of the time!

The wiring is such that the first chakra draws closer to the second chakra, joining with it.

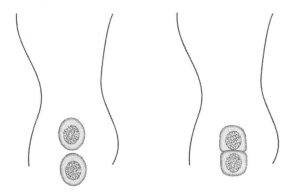

So our first task in opening the second chakra is to identify it as separate from the base!

We make space between them?

Exactly. Let's first try making some physical space between them. Lie on a cushion, the edge of a bed, or a block so that the edge of your spine is hanging off the edge of the support.

The exact position does not at all matter. What you are looking for is tension in the spine. What we will do is release tension from both the back and the front of our spine.

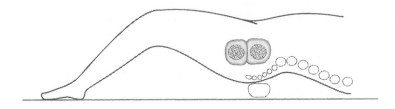

What do you mean by front and back?

Think of the spine and sacrum as a thick cable with a down side and also an up side.

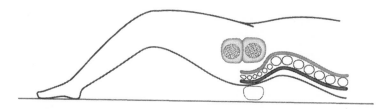

We will use the breath to release first the bottom, and then the top. The two are actually set to different tensions, and will release differently.

Breathe in and breathe down, curling the back of your sacrum down and over the edge. Breathe in and breathe down, feeling for the new curve.

Keep feeling the curve and feel for the tightness stretching along the top of your sacrum. Breathe in and breathe down, releasing the top line to curl closer to the bottom. Both front and back of the sacrum are now curled over the edge of the support.

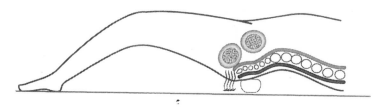

A new and different sensation to explore, isn't it, to feel two different sides of your spine? Keep exploring it with your breath.

If you push downward with your breath, the first chakra will roll over the dangling tip of your spine, as if off a cliff.

When you feel that, you have created space between the first
and second chakras.

Just to explore a bit further, breathe in, and breathe out
the sides of your pelvis. Your pelvis will widen and move as
the muscles relax, seeking a new balance.

Try laying on your side to release the sacrum down to the
ground. This releases the left and right sides of the sacrum.

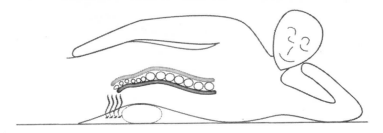

And opening the chakra?

Like the other chakras, we can open the second with the
breath. Come to a comfortable seated position. Breathe in,
and breathe out through your pelvis into the space in front of
you.

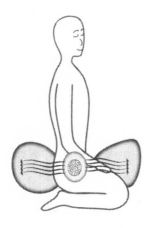

Breathe in, and breathe out through the back of the pelvis. Accommodate the release. It moves things around, doesn't it?

The first chakra now is easy, and we've been working on it all the way through. Simply breathe in and breathe down. Feel the rebound of energy up through your now more open spine and energy channels. It's like opening a door in a hallway: it's only when you open both doors that you feel the breeze!

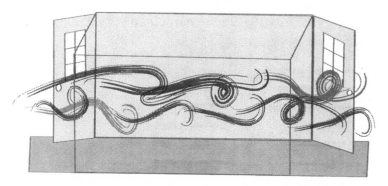

So our chakras are now tuned?

We've only tuned them all once! There are no miracles in Tantra, only exploration. Keep exploring all your chakras and they will become tuned in the best way possible for YOU.

12 The why of antenna repair

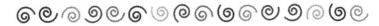

What does tuning our chakras achieve?

Most of us live our lives in a state of confusion. We are confused as to who we are, who other people are. We are confused about how we feel about our families. We enter into relationships with other people because they feel good, or because they satisfy some itch or need we have. We may be able to identify how it feels good, but how often do we identify *why* it feels good?

It's not wrong to simply say "This feels good on a deep level, and I'm going to go with the feeling." There are times when we can't see clearly, but have to feel our way through things.

But if our chakras, our energy centers, are clouded by old patterns and behaviors, we can misread the signals we get from the universe and the humans we encounter.

Not being able to see clearly, we fall back on whatever patterns worked for us in the past. That can set us up for some painful lessons.

In what way?

Let's say we meet someone that we find very attractive. We feel good around them, their energy complements our own, we connect with them on certain levels. It's almost as if there is a mirror between us, some parts of which are clear, some

reflect back to us only what we prefer to see. We do not look
carefully at who they really are, we simply assume that if we
feel good with them on some frequencies, everything will be
fine.

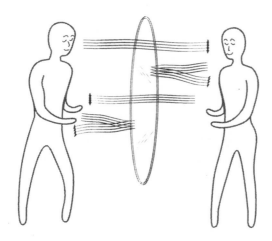

For a while we may be content. If we notice that they do
not always treat other people well, we excuse it by saying that
they are thrifty, or reserved, or shy, or impatient with stupidity.
When the day comes that they do not treat us well, we are
shocked. And we say "I should have known…"

We did know, but we wanted to satisfy our own needs, so
we didn't take the time to see clearly enough that the fit wasn't
going to work.

Most of us learn a lesson from this. But if we are running
strong patterns and have invested a lot of energy into the
relationship, we may feel betrayed, blame them, and run back
out to find someone else to satisfy that same pattern.

If we can see clearly after the fact why it didn't work, we
will choose far better next time.

If we see clearly enough in the beginning, our choices will
be much better and much more satisfying.

So how does one see clearly?

Seeing clearly is a matter of fine-tuning your perception to see more clearly your own patterns, and the patterns of the world. It is a matter of increasing the sensitivity, the awareness, of your internal energy antenna.

Antenna?

Why should we have this ability to feel and project energy? Why should we melt at some things and stiffen at others? Why should charismatic movie stars like Greta Garbo, performers like Luciano Pavarotti, or politicians (name one!) touch chords in us?

All for the same reason: we interact with the world, constantly giving and receiving energy. We are alert to currents coming our way, and we pass them along to others. We are affected by the energy we receive from others and we affect others with the energy we send out.

Giving and receiving energy...

We talked earlier about how the mechanistic view of the universe is outdated. Modern systems theory sees everything, including humans, not as separate pieces, but as open systems that take in energy from the environment and put energy back into the environment.

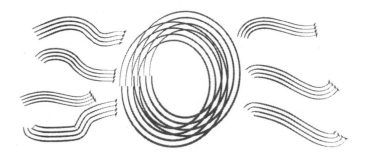

The energy we receive comes in so many ways: sunshine, the energy stored in food, the invisible cosmic radiation passing through our bodies. All of these energies are part of our lives, and so, too, is the energy we receive from other humans.

Human energy.

Of course! We love, we hate, we embrace, we reject. And all these things happen in turn to us. If everything in the universe is energy, and humans are made of energy, what else could it be that we exchange with others?

Some energy exchanges are direct with other humans: family, friends, lovers, shopkeepers. There are cultural energy currents as well: religion, music, fashion, stories, and attitudes toward just about everything. Since the creation of the Internet, cultural energy/information flows much faster through humans. The Internet is new wiring for human society.

Why should we see everything as energy?

Well, mostly because everything IS energy. We can't deny it, we can't fight it, we might as well accept it and go on from there!

What's wrong with the way we look at the world now?

Nothing, really. Except that it doesn't work any more. We need more flexible concepts based on our latest understanding of the universe to help us navigate through life.

Centuries ago, people believed the world was flat. That was fine, for the most part, because few people needed to know that it wasn't.

Today, you can't live fully in the world if you insist on believing it is flat and that the ocean runs off the edge. It isn't flat, and that's all there is to it. Talking and behaving as if the earth is flat is too limiting.

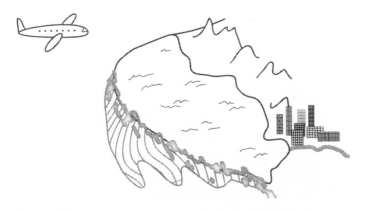

Talking and behaving as if everything is separate from each other is also too limiting. Seeing the world and everything in it as patterns of energy gives us terrific new tools for understanding who we are, and how we live in the world.

Such as?

A good example is the *butterfly effect*, the idea that the fluttering of a butterfly's wings could lead to a tornado somewhere else in the world. The idea comes from new concepts about open energy systems and non-linear processes. It makes sense to us that small events could have unpredictably large effects.

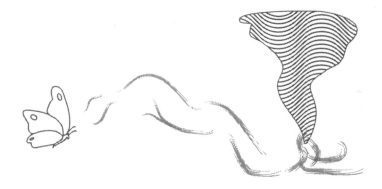

Let's go back to our neglected antennas.

Okay, back to antennas...

If we see that thoughts, emotions, feelings are made of energy, we can see how people send them out to us and how we send them back. We are, if you will, antennas that pick up frequencies. We can focus on just one person, we can take in the feel of a street scene at a glance, we can also stretch wide to feel as much of the world as we can, like lying on the grass and drinking in the blue sky.

Just like our giant scientific telescopes have multiple mirrors and receivers, we do too in our own bodies. Our chakras are the mirrors on our antenna. We have already explored how to open them when we breathed out the front and back of each of them. Let's run through them again.

Seat yourself comfortably, breathe in, and breathe down.

Breathe in and breathe out through the front and then through the back, of each energy center. It doesn't matter which one you start with or what order you follow. Not if you do all of them!

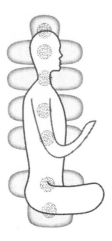

Now for the sending and receiving part.

Sending and receiving...

This is lovely to do with another person, but it also works with a mirror. Stand or sit in front of a mirror so that your head and chest are visible.

Look at yourself in the mirror. Let your vision rest on the right side of the face in the mirror. Gaze at the eye on the right side.

Breathe in, and breathe down. Breathe in, and with your out-breath let the left side of your head relax. Look at the eye on the right with the whole left side of your head. The left side of your head will feel connected to the right side of the image in the mirror.

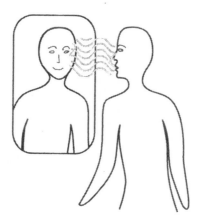

Switch your gaze to the eye on the left of the image. Breathe in and breathe down. Breathe in, and let the whole right side of your head relax and gaze at the mirror.

When this relaxation becomes quite comfortable, move your gaze down the mirror to your chest. Breathe in, and breathe out from your chest to its reflection in the mirror.

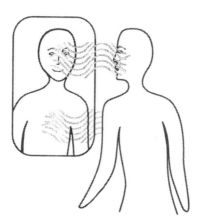

If you can do this with your own reflection, imagine what it is like to move through your day, sending and receiving energy with everyone you meet!

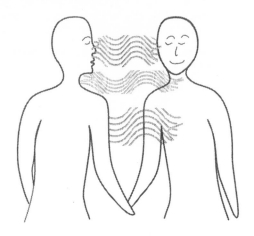

Is this a trick?

Maybe, if you think of your image in the mirror as a construct of your own mind. But it really doesn't matter, because if we can send energy out from our mind and heart to a mirror and back, we can certainly send it out to other people!

13 Balancing opposites

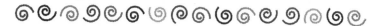

Opposites? I thought you suggested that duality didn't exist...

It's all in your perspective. Duality is like particles and waves, energy and information: two different ways of looking at the same thing. Duality is contrast: sharpen the contrast so gray becomes black and white.

The contrast of duality is a very useful tool. But there are other tools, as well. Sometimes we work with opposites, sometimes we balance them, sometimes we merge them.

Working with opposites means...

Just that we use them. We use them to decide bad and good, left or right, up or down, marry this one or that one. Life works that way sometimes, and when it does, we choose one or the other.

When do we choose something else?

Whenever we need to, which is much or maybe most of the time. We should always check, before accepting two options, to see if there's a third way. Finding truth falls into this category. When you hear from two people opposite sides of the same story, the truth is always a third story.

That's when we balance them?

That's usually the next thing we try. We balance the opposites in different ways: we balance them in our mind against facts we discover, we balance them in our heart by what we think of the people involved.

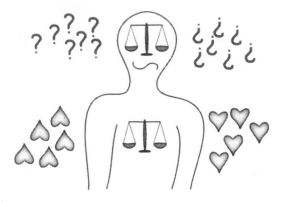

Often we balance them unconsciously with multiple chakras. How many times in our life have any of us said of some situation, "This feels a little off to me?" We may not be sure why, but we're picking up some energy that doesn't feel right!

And when we can't balance them?

We tip to one side or another, like scales. But we CAN balance them, and often we can even merge them so that they are not separate, but merely two sides of the same coin.

How?

Let's start by first grabbing hold of two opposites. Think of someone you love who has passed on. Think of how sad you are that they are gone.

But there is happiness here, too. The First Law of Thermodynamics (heat/energy flow) states that energy may neither be created or destroyed, only changed. If we are made of energy and that energy cannot be destroyed, then does it matter if we are here in this body on this planet, or out in the greater flow of the universe? Does it matter after we pass on whether we stay in roughly the same pattern or are spread through the beauty of the universe?

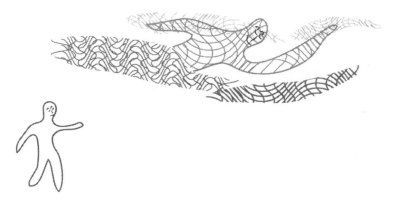

Think of how happy you are that they are now joyful in the universe and no longer bound by their pains or sorrows.

Hold your hands in front of you palms upward. In your left hand place your sorrow at their passing. Feel the weight of it in your hand.

In your right hand place your happiness. Breathe in, and breathe down, finding a still point to rest. Let your hands simply hold the two feelings.

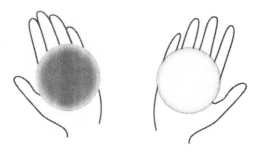

Breathe in, and breathe out through your heart. And
realize that you are the connection between the two feelings.

You are the connection between the two feelings.

It's not a bad way to look at it. Because we not only feel
the two sides, we can connect them.

Breathe in, and breathe down, centering yourself. Slowly
turn your palms toward each other and begin to bring your
hands together. It may feel as if there is resistance, or if the
space between your hands is thick. Keep breathing, and with
every breath bring them a little closer.

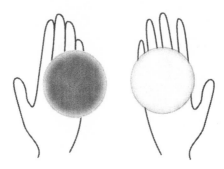

You can merge the two feelings by using your hands to feel
the space in the middle, or using your sight to see one space
with two hands rather than two hands each with something in

it. If it helps, draw a line in your mind from one hand to the other.

How you connect them doesn't matter. When you do it, there will be a lessening of tension, and the two opposites will feel like two sides of the same thing.

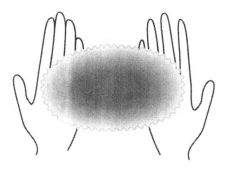

For good measure, let's get the heart chakra involved. Breathe in, and breathe out through your heart into the space between your hands.

Words cannot describe this. When you are ready, breathe in, and breathe out, releasing your hands.

14 The butterfly effect

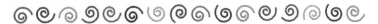

That's where a butterfly can cause a tornado...

Not quite. The term *butterfly effect* means that a small action in one place can set into motion a pattern of events. In turn, this pattern merges with others to cause a major effect somewhere else. The pattern is unpredictable; it doesn't follow a straight line.

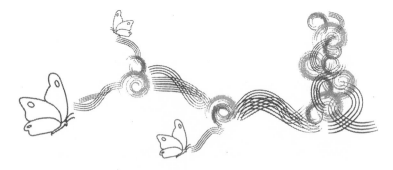

This *non-linear* sequence is a big change in thinking from classical science.

Non-linear...

Before the 20th century, scientific thinking was mostly concerned with processes that seemed to run in a straight line. Due to the work of scientists like Sir Isaac Newton, a way of looking at the world emerged that suggested that actions and reactions were regular and predictable. You always got the same result from the same experiment. Processes ran forwards and backwards and time was reversible. Every action had an equal and opposite reaction. You couldn't get more out of a system than you put in.

Newtonian mechanics is a good tool for learning things that are very regular, like machines, but it is far from the truth for most everything else!

Why?

Newtonian mechanics deals with simple, closed systems. We know today, however, that almost everything in the universe is a *complex* system, an open system, where energy flows in, is processed, and flows back out. Plants are a good example. Plants take in sunshine and water and nutrients, grow themselves, and give back oxygen and water.

Plants are complex systems, and you can't predict the evolution of a plant just from the raw materials. It doesn't grow in a straight line.

How things grow in non-linear ways was discovered as a result of research into the Second Law of Thermodynamics. The Second Law says that energy always flows from regions of more energy to regions of less energy. This is popularly known as *entropy*, and has been interpreted to mean that the universe will run down to a state where everything is uniform, lifeless, and cold.

The only problem with this is that the universe isn't running down but is busy building all kinds of energy systems. A scientist named Ilya Prigogine demonstrated, in open systems he called *dissipative structures*, how evolving systems move from order to chaos to higher order.

Higher order?

Everyone has seen a stream where the water flows smoothly, with hardly a ripple. Let's call this the *steady state*. We think of it as well-ordered.

When the stream reaches rocks, it breaks up into what looks like chaos, tumbling all over itself.

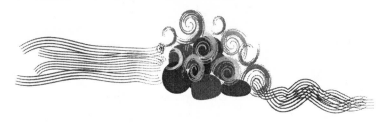

What Prigogine discovered is that what looks like chaos isn't. The water has acquired enough energy to reach a higher, more complex energy state. A more complex information state. There is more going on in the rapids than in the quiet stream! More interactions, more energy flows.

Prigogine found that at the moment turbulence or chaos disrupts the balance of the system, the system can go in one of two directions. One direction is to shed the energy, drop to a lower energy state, and return to an smooth flow. The other direction is to incorporate the energy and emerge with more complex patterns that can handle the increased energy. Prigogine called this *jumping* to a new, higher energy state.

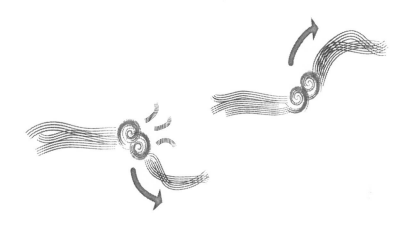

Is there only up or down?

In the systems Prigogine studied, there was either up or there was down. But in other systems there may well be a sideways!

There are several interesting things about this process.

The first is that there is no way to predict whether a system will move up or down. All of the rules that worked for the nice, orderly flow don't work when the system has to jump higher or lower. Prigogine called the point at which the system jumps the *bifurcation point*, because the system has to go up or down. At the bifurcation point, the rules disappear, and a chance event (like a butterfly!) can cause the system to go one way or the other. Let's call it the *butterfly point*.

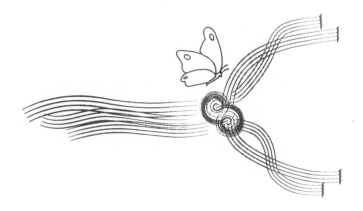

So at the butterfly point, where the system has to do something with the extra energy, a chance event can cause the system to jump in one direction or the other.

The second interesting thing about this process is that complex systems are more likely to jump to higher levels of energy and complexity than to lower levels. Once a system begins to jump higher, it jumps faster and faster, the pace accelerating.

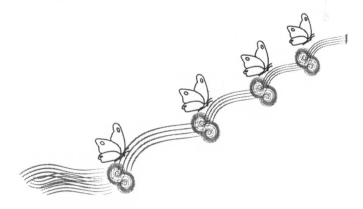

The third interesting thing is that the nature of the jump depends on where the system has been. You can't leap from cave paintings to quantum mechanics in one step. Your history and direction help determine the possibilities.

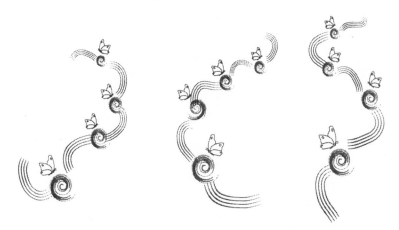

A fourth interesting thing is that you cannot predict when a butterfly point will occur. There is no way to tell from the relatively deterministic processes in the steady state when they will fail to cope with new information and cause the system to hit a butterfly point.

How about some examples?

Historians have argued for the last couple centuries about whether history is determined by great movements or by individuals. It makes a lot of sense that during times of relative calm, individuals can't do much to sway the whole system.

But it is precisely at the butterfly point that an individual like a Julius Caesar can make a big difference. Enough to cause the divided Roman Republic of his time to become the Mediterranean-spanning Roman Empire.

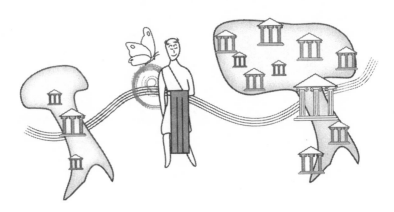

A different example would be the Great Potato Famine in Ireland in the nineteenth century. The combination of land distribution and failure of the potato crops caused a crisis. Ireland shed energy in the form of people who migrated all over the world. Ireland dropped to a lower, less turbulent, energy level.

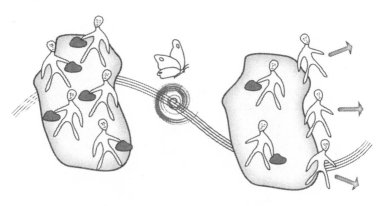

An example of the pace of change (jumping) might be the entire history of the last couple centuries! As the world has become more and more complex, it is hitting butterfly points faster, and jumping faster to new states and more complexity.

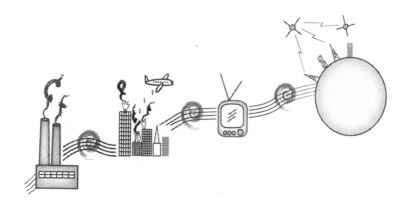

This happens in our own lives, too. We all have periods where not much seems to happen and we do the same thing day after day. If a new person or activity or idea comes into our life we change to accommodate it, often jumping to places that surprise us when we look backward. When the old patterns don't work any more, even a chance remark can set us off in a new direction!

So our world is made up of order and chaos, chance and complexity?

Yes, and all of these things are going on at the same time. In our work life we might be steady state, even while our personal life is falling apart and our social life is changing dramatically. You can probably find many examples in your own life of order and chaos, chance, and increasing complexity.

Life sounds very confusing!

It might seem that way, but these new ways of looking at the world clear up many things we haven't understood.

We know now that evolution is a basic process of the universe, and that evolving energy systems can change quickly.

We understand now how people and societies can blossom, how small changes can lead to major shifts.

We know that we are not trapped in our current patterns forever. That we never know when a butterfly point may occur and we will jump to new levels of energy and awareness.

We know that we can choose to deny new energy/information coming our way; we can retreat to lower energy levels. We all know people who do this, and hold on tenaciously to outmoded ideas and behavior.

We know that we can choose to embrace new energy, and lead richer lives as a result.

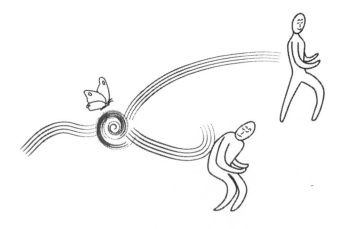

We know that our actions in every moment count, because in that moment we might well BE the butterfly.

And we know that order and chaos are integral parts of the same process and that both are necessary for us to grow.

If life often seems to you like a roller coaster ride, just remember that the direction is still up!

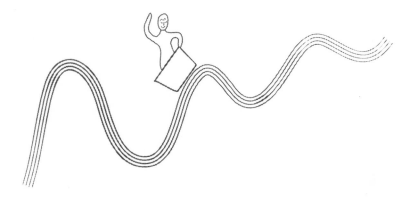

Note on Science:

Dr. Ilya Prigogine was awarded the Nobel Prize in 1977 for his work on dissipative structures. His work was founded on the discoveries of many eminent scientists before him.

Dr. Prigogine was well aware of, and wrote about, the wider implications of his work. Erich Jantsch went on to describe humans as dissipative systems in a creative, dissipative universe.

The interpretation here extends further than Dr. Prigogine's writings.

15 Up or down, or sideways

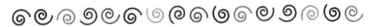

You implied that you can *choose* up or down at the butterfly point...

Yes. Ilya Prigogine suggested that a very complex system could choose its own direction. Let's switch to an information perspective to see how.

When a tree grows, enduring drought, bugs, freezes, and floods, the history of that tree, the information of what happened to that tree, is written in the growth rings.

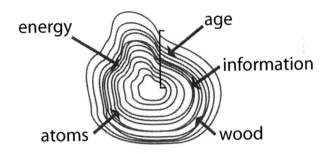

When we look at tree rings, what we see depends on how we look: atoms, molecules, energy patterns, information. A very complex system has an enormous amount of information about its past conditions and its current condition. As a tree evolves, the options for growth are limited by its wiring, its history and its ability to change.

So, too with humans. Except that we process energy differently, we remake ourselves much more quickly. We may not know exactly how conscious trees are and how much choice they have, but we do know about humans!

So we can choose up or down?

Yes. Sometime consciously, sometimes unconsciously. There are times we swirl all unknowing into the new, and times we consciously choose to step up and change our lives. Sometimes we unconsciously deflect energy that would change us, and at other times we consciously say a defiant *No!* and literally push it away or retreat sideways. The very sad case is when someone retreats to a much earlier and lower pattern of energy and never emerges again from it.

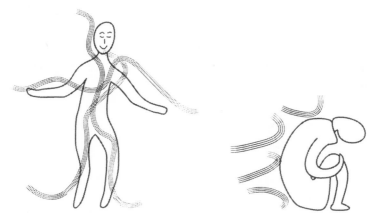

There are middle options, too. Humans are much more complicated than scientific models, and they are self-aware systems that can choose a direction. Much of the time humans keep things familiar, accepting some new energy and deflecting other new energy.

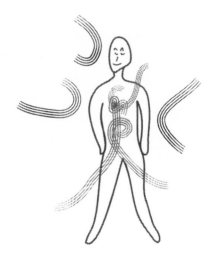

How do we choose?

Remember that the body is an evolving wave pattern of energy/information. This is not just an image; it is our latest understanding of what we are.

We absorb energy into our wave pattern from everything we encounter, all the energy that flows around us. When we absorb this energy/information, we incorporate it into our evolving pattern, the way a child absorbs language and uses it to communicate.

If we are unaware of our own patterns, the energy finds whatever channels are already there. The energy is absorbed by the channel and reinforces the channel. Day to day living is a good example. Much of our life is about doing the same things every day. That's why we go on vacation!

The daily things we do run through the same channels over and over. Like water, in time they carve the channels deeper. So deep that we cannot imagine being without them.

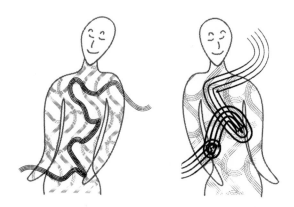

Whether our channels are supple or deep-carved, large amounts of energy create turbulence in them.

Like the stream and the rapids?

Yes, very much so. When the energy is below a certain amount it just becomes part of the flow of the stream. If the energy is more than the stream can absorb into its current pattern, the stream becomes turbulent with new currents and whirlpools.

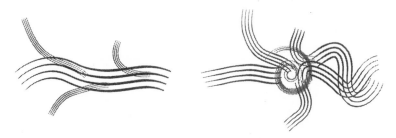

Humans are the same way. New energy will change the current patterns in us, at least for a time. A love affair can make us glow with energy, make everything fresh, change how we see and taste things. After a while, we can decide to keep the new patterns, let them fade, or try to bury them completely.

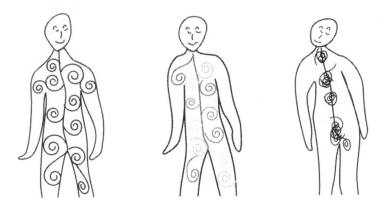

Too much energy, such as in a childhood trauma, may cause us to shift our patterns dramatically. The patterns bend and twist to minimize the damage. They may curl inward to present a face that deflects the energy. They may get crunched hard enough to bend and kink. They may even get shredded and torn.

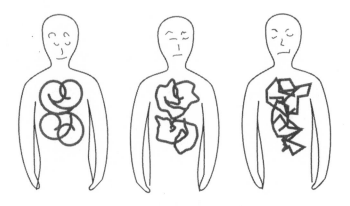

What happens?

Time does! We are not any single moment in time, but an evolving pattern. However we are affected by the energy we take in, we continue to evolve because we live in time. So in time, the three patterns we just looked at will change and grow.

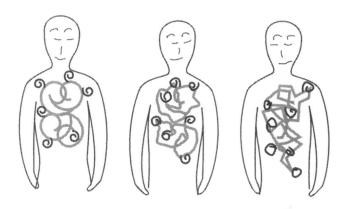

People branch out from wherever they are as more new experiences and energy is added to their lives over time. Some people may try to stay the same, but the universe does not flow in such a way that we can either stay in one place or move backward, as much as we might wish to. We encounter butterfly points all the time, where we must choose how to respond.

But how do we choose at the butterfly point?

First by noticing the energy flow. When you get hit by a big wave at the beach, you know it immediately. There is no choice, you have to do something!

You can retreat into your body, hoping to ride out being pummeled by the wave until you can re-establish control.

You can throw yourself against the wave, trying to match its strength and ride it out.

Or you can stretch your awareness into both the wave and your body at the same time.

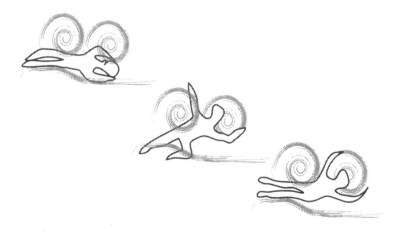

Stretch your awareness?

Yes, that's the next thing you do. And it's something we can actually do quite well.

When the wave hits, you can try to feel for the way it is moving, and fit your body into it a little more comfortably. With your body a little more relaxed, and with more awareness of what is happening around you, there is another moment to again feel and react.

Another example might be slipping on steps. If all you are focused on is the feeling in the pit of your stomach, you are just waiting to hit bottom. You can try to throw yourself in some other direction and hopefully avoid injury. Or you can try to sense where your body is in relation to the ground, and change the tension in your body to spread out the impact. In the meantime, of course, looking for something to grab on to!

Isn't this just part of living?

Absolutely! This extending our awareness happens whether we notice it or not. We have reptilian, primate, and human patterns in our bodies that reach out to the world and respond. But are we paying attention, or just using reflexes that we created earlier in our lives?

How would we know?

Simply by exploring our own patterns. Seeing what there is to see. Feeling what there is to feel. When you find a pattern in your body, in your emotions, in your thoughts, there is an unmistakable recognition. After all, it IS a part of you.

Let's try some stretching we did earlier, but this time from a different perspective.

Lie on your side with the top leg stretched forward and the top arm stretched backward.

The exact position is not important. When we did this earlier we were looking for tension. This time we will look for the pattern of tension in the position.

Twist your body so that there is tension along the whole line of the twist.

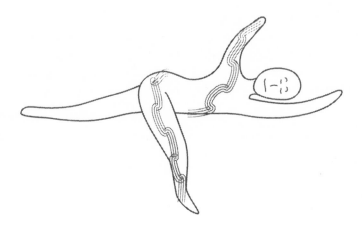

Hold the position in tension. If you need to release a little of it, breathe in, and breathe down a little.

Where do you feel the tension the most? The head, the shoulder, the chest, the ribs? Or is it further down in the hips or the outside of the leg?

Choose the place with the greatest tension, and while holding the tension in the rest of the line, breathe in, and breathe down, releasing just the chosen area.

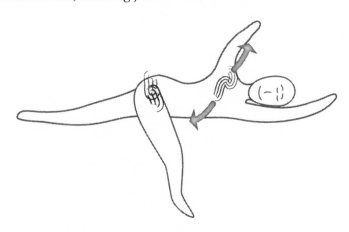

What does the pattern of tension feel like now? It will certainly feel different. And another area of your body will now feel the most tension.

Choose that area, breathe in, and release just that area.

Explore your body position, releasing areas, moving around to find new lines of tension in your back, shoulder blades, neck, pelvis.

Notice how different positions create different patterns of tension. And how every movement creates a new pattern of tension.

Observing patterns while working with them is shaking out the blanket with exquisite attention!

16 Left and right, together again

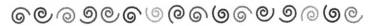

Left and right together?

We are so used to having a left side and a right side! They are different from each other, and we use them differently. And they can differ greatly from one human to the next. Left-handed people and right-handed people use their hands and bodies differently.

A right-handed person might use the right side for mobility and fine-tuning, for reaching out and manipulating something. The left side would be used more for balance and stability, anchoring the right side while it explores things. There is no right side without the left!

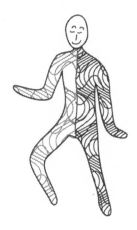

They work together.

Yes. How do YOUR left and right sides work together? Let's explore this.

Lie down on your left side, with the bottom leg and arm bent for stability and comfort. Breathe in, and breathe down, relaxing the bottom side.

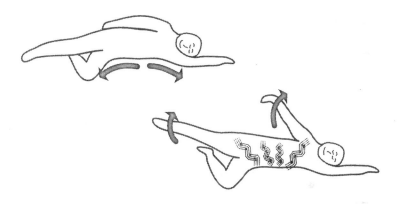

Raise your top arm and leg. Feel how your bottom side braces and supports the movement of the top side. Move your top arm and leg. Where does the bottom side tense up to support the motion? Which movements are graceful? Which ones feel ungraceful?

Stretch your arm and leg in front of you, letting them drop to the surface you are lying on. Stretch forward with the arm and leg until you can feel tension along your spine.

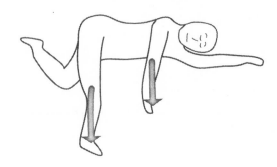

Breathe in, and breathe down, releasing the tension.

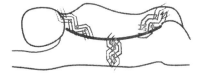

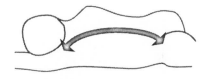

What does this new position feel like? Does your spine move more freely?

Switch sides. How does this side feel different from the first? And it does feel different, doesn't it?

Yes, the two sides feel different.

That is because you use them differently, move them differently. They have developed different patterns of muscles and tension.

We can see this in a mirror. Stand naturally and comfortably in front of a mirror. Breathe in, and breathe down, relaxing and straightening. Where are your feet? Are they facing straight forward, or is one or both turned out?

Chances are one foot is turned out (pointed outward) more than the other. If the foot is turned out, then so is the leg. And that means the pelvis is turned out, as well.

You can check this by pointing the outward-turned foot to the center. Bring your head back up (you *were* looking at your feet, weren't you?). Breathe in, and breathe down, relaxing your body. When you relax, your body will turn slightly in the direction of the foot that was turned out, and you will be looking slightly off to the side.

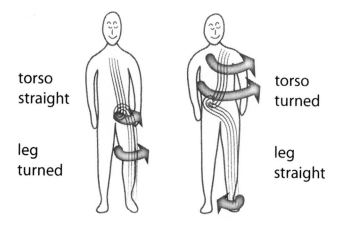

torso
straight

leg
turned

torso
turned

leg
straight

Why?

Few of us live in a body that is perfectly balanced. Our pelvis or shoulders may be twisted, or one side may be higher than the other.

Isn't everyone different?

Yes, of course. But the human body is designed so that if everything is in balance, your feet, your pelvis and your body will be pointing straight forward, and you will be looking straight ahead. It was the insight of Ida Rolf, the creator of a body-straightening technique called *rolfing*, that being balanced was the most energy-efficient posture for the body. If your posture is not in balance, you are spending energy to stay that way!

Because...

Your body has adjusted to trauma or disease or learned patterns of movement. You have shifted tension in the body over time to compensate for being unbalanced, and you are spending energy to maintain that tension.

So we have to re-balance the body?

First we have to recognize the imbalances, and see if we can understand why the imbalance has occurred. Sometimes it can lie deep in our childhood.

Everyone, unfortunately, has seen a child who cringes away when feeling threatened. If you are that child, and are right-handed, you might always turn to your right, presenting your left side and shielding your right side.

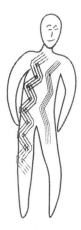

Over time, your body will strengthen the patterns, the muscles, that allow you to make that move quickly. The pelvis may turn so that you always have a little protection on your favored side. You may even develop the habit of keeping people on your left!

We talked earlier about a young plant that is stepped on and recovers, but doesn't quite grow the same way. Humans often have the same experience.

So how do we re-balance?

You do the best you can. There is no one way. Some types of bodywork may be useful in re-aligning your body, but ultimately we have to explore our patterns of movement and posture. Pay attention to how you sit, stand or walk. Play with the way you walk, changing the way you put your foot down, or the pace of your steps.

Notice your habitual movements. Switch some motions from left to right and back again, to see the difference. Notice the difference between your left and right sides. Work them separately and together.

That will re-balance us?

In several ways. It will re-balance you physically over time. It will also improve your motor control and coordination.

Stretching out your patterns will loosen old kinks and connections. The energy will flow more freely in both sides, and will be more available for your use.

More available?

When you are spending energy maintaining a pattern in your body, it is busy and not available for other things. That's why rigid people seem so locked up: their energy is so busy maintaining their tension that they have little to spare for you!

Remember that there is no difference between the physical, mental, emotional and energetic. They are all energy, just in different patterns and using different frequencies. As you loosen the patterns, everything gets loosened up: your body, your energy, your mind, and the emotions you attached to long-ago events.

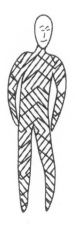 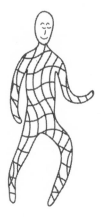

The less energy you have tied up in maintaining old patterns, the more you will have available for everything new coming your way.

Are there exercises?

All of the ones we've explored so far are good, if you bring this added awareness of patterns to them. Everyone's body is different; you must create your own path to your own awareness and balance.

A key part of the body to pay attention to is your pelvis. Most of us think of our pelvis as being fixed, like a single piece in a puzzle. But like the rest of our body, it is tensile, has a left and right side, and we can stretch it and bend it. All of us admire the easy sway of hips. It is not just a movement like a pendulum, it is a dance of many lines of energy.

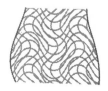 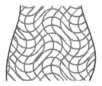

To begin to feel the structure and movement of the pelvis, sit comfortably cross-legged on the floor, a pillow, or a bed. Pull the sides of your pelvis out a little, creating a better base.

Breathe in, and breathe down, letting your sit bones drop. Twist your torso to one side, using your arms to brace the twist. Where do you feel tension?

Breathe in and breathe down, release the tension and let your spine move. It will sway in the direction of the twist.

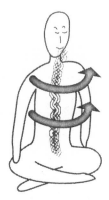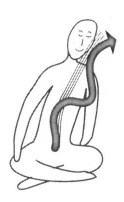

Try a couple different twists, each time breathing in and then breathing down to release the tension.

Now that the upper portion is loose, we can focus our attention on the pelvis. Instead of bracing our arms to twist the torso, we will brace them to twist the pelvis.

Start to twist your body, but resist the twist, braced with your arms. This will transfer the tension to the pelvis. When you can feel the tension in your pelvis, breathe in and breathe down, and release the tension. Your pelvis will move in the opposite direction from the twist. You can feel the left and right sides of your pelvis move in different directions!

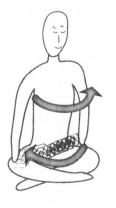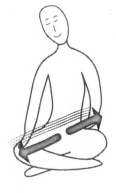

Try as many variations as you like. Once you begin to get the feel for tension in the pelvis, you can reach for it in almost any position. The side-lying positions are especially good for working different sides of the pelvis, and loosening the lower spine and sacrum.

We ought to be able to flex our pelvis in three dimensions. It's designed that way! It is the crossroads of the energy patterns in our body, connecting left to right, up to down.

17 The energy of pain

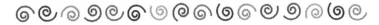

What do you mean by the *energy* of pain?

Pain and pleasure are names we give to certain kinds of sensations, of energy patterns, in our bodies. They definitely get our attention!

So much so that you find them everywhere in human history, art, culture and ceremony. They are inscribed in carvings on temples, initiation rites, painting, sculptures, novels, and poems. They are so much a part of our lives that we simply take them as they are.

But what are they, and why are they so powerful?

Research suggests that the body feels a stimulus and our brains interpret it as pain or pleasure. When we feel pain or pleasure, what we actually feel is not a single stimulus, but a pattern of stimulation. It takes place not just in the body or the head, but in both places.

When you bang your knee, the knee says *Ouch!*

The mind says *Ouch!*

The knee says *Ouch!*

The mind says *Ouch!*

The knee says *Ouch!*

The mind says *Wow! My knee hurts!*

The conversation rockets back and forth so fast we often don't notice the transitions.

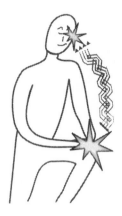

Few people get through life without injury or pain. The pain can be superficial skin agony like sunburn or a scrape. It can be an unbearable itch. Or something so intense in one single part of your body that your head explodes in agony. That's why we often talk of "seeing stars" when our bodies are shocked. We often see stars during orgasm, too.

We are not made of pieces. We are open energy systems that take in energy from our surroundings, incorporate it in some fashion, and send some of it back out again. The energy coming in is the stimulus, the processing is perception of it as pain or pleasure.

How do we process it?

We're hard-wired for sensing pain and reacting to it, so much so that we have short-circuits, or maybe better described as quick-circuits, that relay the pain quicker than our regular nervous system and brains can process, and produce very fast reactions. Most of us can move our hands away from a hot surface before we have time to think about it.

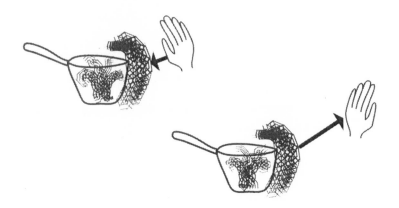

We have quick-circuits for more than pain, we have them for threats, too. When we hear a sound behind us, our hips are already turning, and flashing an impulse to the brain to turn around and pay attention. By the time our head whips around, we are alert and straining for more information.

Are threat and pain similar?

Yes, in that they are things that cause us to pay attention. Threats cause us to pay attention to something outside us. Pain is the body's cry for us to pay attention to something inside us. Pain and threat are an irritation, mild or strong, of our circuits. Any irritation, repeated enough, becomes painful.

And pain and pleasure...

Are quite similar. If we can describe pain as an irritation, we perhaps can describe pleasure as excitation leading to release.

We can see this in our breathing patterns when we experience pleasure. Whether it is the caress of a hand, the pleasure of a good book or a beautiful painting, we almost always tighten, and then release.

When we sigh with pleasure we increase the tension on the rib cage and then deliciously release it.

Try sighing a few times. Notice your torso: the pattern will be stiffen, release, stiffen, release. Not all that different from pain and the cessation of pain. How often we feel a great sense of pleasure when the pain goes away!

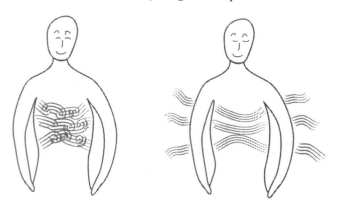

Everyone feels pain and pleasure differently; the same stimulus one person interprets as pleasure can be interpreted by someone else as pain. Pleasure in one moment can become pain in another if the excitement becomes irritating. And pain can become pleasure if it leads to excitement and release.

The difference between pain and pleasure is in degree and intent. But let's stick with pain for now: the intensity and the effect have a great impact on us.

How?

The intensity of pain can make some pretty big dents in us! We know this instinctively, but we can also test this in our own bodies.

Think about a pain you have experienced.

How close can you get to feeling it again?

Is your body tightening up as you get close to that feeling?

The dents in our patterns caused by pain yell at us whenever we go near them. Our bodies never forget, and stay on guard just in case it should ever happen again.

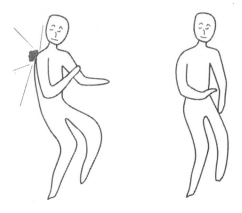

Stay on guard?

Like trees, our energy patterns reflect the things that happen to us. We grow around it, but the imprint is still there.

When we hurt something anywhere in our energy system, the system rallies around the hurt place. We relax some muscles to ease the strain, tighten others to take up the slack. Our bodies heal and re-balance themselves, at least as best they can, unless we get in our own way.

How do we get in the way?

By running patterns that keep the irritation going, that feed the pain and keep it alive.

We're complex creatures, and we learn along the way what our most effective strategies for survival are. We may learn to focus on the pain and complain about it loudly so that

someone else will take care of us. We might learn to linger
with it, so people will take care of us longer. We might learn
to enhance it, running energy through the pain pattern, so our
complaints are more believable.

Some people might learn to keep quiet and try to heal
themselves, so that they do not show weakness to others.
Others will do their best to ignore the pain, so that they do
not show weakness to themselves. Most of us use all of these
strategies in varying mixtures.

That's understandable, but does pain really last that long?

What if you didn't know how to live without it? What
if the trauma was so great, or so repeated, that your whole
system reorganized itself around the pain?

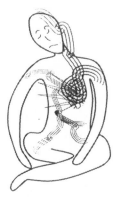

It happens. I met a woman who had been in a car accident
three years earlier. She was in pain, she was knotted and
twisted, and moved awkwardly. When she got on the table for
a massage she was so tight that her arms and legs were stuck
upward. During a massage that released a lot of tension, she
suddenly took a deep breath and relaxed completely.

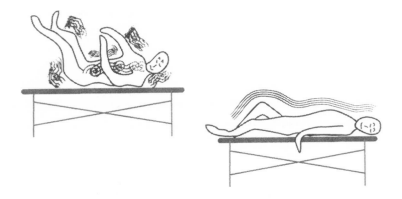

She stopped radiating pain. After a few moments of trance, she refocused, and her body returned to its locked-up state.

The relaxation showed that there was no physiological reason for her body to be cramped and hurting. She had just had enough of a shock that she no longer knew what to do when she wasn't focused on the pain.

Was the pain real?

If you were locked up all the time, you'd be in pain, too!

The original pain was real, the current pain is real. But the current pain is being sustained by the energy put into it.

This is a dramatic example, but all of us know people who are wrapped around their pain. We can stay wrapped around a pain for decades after it happened. And we try many different ways of dealing with old pain until somewhere along the way we stretch it out and let some of the tension go.

How do you get focused on pain?

A good visual might be what happens when you bring a flame too close to the edge of an unfurling flower petal. The energy from the flame disrupts the pattern of the petal, which is not built to handle that much energy.

The petal blackens and curls, an outward manifestation of the chemical oxidation and disrupted structural patterns in the petal.

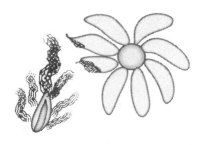

If the damage is slight, the petal may keep growing, but with some permanently changed edges. If the damage is greater, the petal may abandon that area and simply grow in another direction. If the damage is severe, the whole petal may be affected and die after a while, unable to regain a workable balance.

The flower petal is a simple example. Think of how complex humans are, how many energy centers we have. How we can choose what direction to grow ourselves, how we can tighten our patterns to shut the world out. We have many choices as to how to proceed from a traumatic, or a not-so-traumatic, event.

Then why do people run the same patterns?

If you have pain, it may seem a better bargain to stick with what you know rather than take a chance on acquiring more!

Everybody has pain. That was the great insight of the Buddha, that life is suffering, a teaching that strikes a chord in billions of humans. Why else should we want to believe in a paradise?

So life is suffering?

Pain is necessary, suffering is optional! Suffering is how you handle pain. And you can choose your approach.

When you sprain your ankle, the pain tells you to avoid pressure on it. One approach is to try to ignore the pain and walk normally. You are impatient for it to heal. That often results in further injury and a trip to the doctor. And you probably shoot it dirty looks every time it hurts!

Another approach is to take all the pressure off it by grabbing a crutch and hobbling around. You'll get tired of this and give your ankle long-suffering looks. The ankle will heal in a different position than it had when it was supporting you, and you will need to work with it or have to walk differently.

A third approach is to work with the injury as soon as it happens. Testing different pressures on it, testing the range of motion. Learning to walk slowly and deliberately rather than at your normal pace. You can control the amount of pain by paying exquisite attention to how much pressure you put on it. You will look at your foot in relation to the ground and to obstacles.

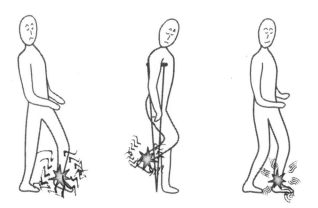

In this third way, you actually participate in healing your ankle, rather than being impatient with it or waiting for it to heal. You change the pace and style of your walk, change the pressure on the ankle, rest and exercise all the muscles. Paying exquisite attention to it will help it heal! And you may just wind up with a better, more flexible ankle than you had before.

There is pain in life, but it is an opportunity to grow in ways we wouldn't have thought of, and learn things we wouldn't think to look for when not in pain.

How do we look for pain?

You don't have to look for it, you just have to notice it! Pain is a heightened energy/information state. When cells are under tension, they radiate that information. The more tension, the louder the yelling. Right up to the moment of disruption, of death.

Pain creates a whole pattern of tension, and we can release it by working from the outside lesser tension to the greater tension underneath.

Any exercise will do, but let's try a new one focused on the spine.

Find an object to lay down on. A fist-sized rubber ball filled with sand would be perfect, but look for something not too big, not too small, not too hard, not too soft. Wrap it in a towel if it has hard edges.

Place the object under your spine above your sacrum and just below the small of your back.

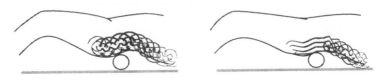

Breathe in, and breathe down. Your muscles will relax and release, your sacrum will drop more firmly onto the ball, and your spine will drop and stretch out.

Feel the new position and the different pressure. You may begin to feel uncomfortable as the ball encounters tighter areas deeper in towards the spine.

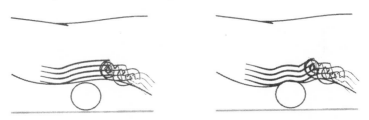

Stretch out this new tension. Breathe in, and breathe down, releasing it. Breathe in, and when you breathe down try to curve your spine over the top of the ball.

Try moving the ball up the spine, releasing one area at a time. When you reach your neck, curl your neck around the object, feeling for tense places and letting them go.

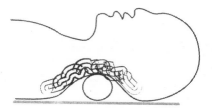

Whenever the tension gets too close to pain, your body will move of its own accord away from it. Go with the motion and re-settle yourself in a more comfortable position and try again.

Pain is a useful guide to deep patterns of tension in our body. The deep, painful places are curled up tight, focused inward.

If we really want to re-tune our antennas and feel more of the energy in the world, we need to deal with the painful places in us that are paying attention only to themselves.

If we have the tools, why not use them?

18 Pleasure is a verb

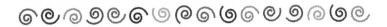

A verb?

Pleasure is not a thing we obtain or possess, it is a pattern of sensation inside us. If pain is a strong irritation of energy, we can think of pleasure as an excitation and release.

Every human is unique and has unique wiring, so the line between pain and pleasure can be almost anywhere. There are people for whom the slightest touch is painful, and people for whom the strongest stimuli are pleasure. Most people, of course, fall somewhere in the middle.

In fact, the habit of falling in the middle is proven science. Many disciplines make use of a bell curve, which represents a statistical model that says that two-thirds of a population will fall inside one standard deviation. In simpler terms, it means that two-thirds of a population will be bunched up in the middle, with fewer on the ends of the curve.

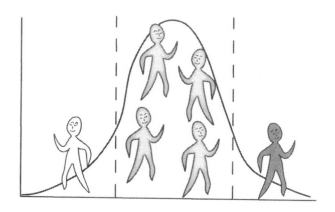

Don't worry if you are on the far side of the curve in anything. Somebody HAS to be!

So differences in feeling pleasure are normal?

To a large extent, yes. But we still make our own choices. Such as what kinds of pleasure to pursue, and how much edge we want.

Edge?

The edge between pleasure and pain, excitation and irritation. People use both pleasure and pain to achieve heightened energy states. Many people explore the edge, pushing it farther out. Pretty soon they're skipping most of the transitions and just pursuing the edge. Looking for the next high of one sort or another, a more intense energy to run through the channels.

The more often you run energy through a channel, the more energy that channel takes in, and the stronger the channel becomes.

Think of the first time someone yelled at you. It was probably pretty shocking, wasn't it? The very first reaction is to be a little stunned, as the energy finds its way through you.

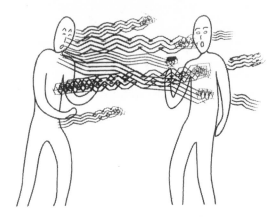

When it happens again, you are better prepared. You now have some channels to handle the energy. You may learn to deflect it, or to run it through the same stress points, hurt points. If you don't walk away at some point, it may become part of your daily routine, a part you don't notice that much anymore. Eventually, you become so used to this exchange of energy that without it, you don't feel quite the same as you usually do.

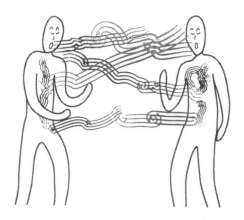

Is yelling a form of pleasure?

It can be, if it involves the increase and release of tension.
Children run around yelling all the time. Remember how
good it felt as a child to yell as loudly as you can? Popular
entertainment throughout history often has lots of yelling and
hitting, from medieval puppet shows to cartoons to football
games.

The pleasure is in the excitation and release of tension.
The amount of tension you prefer for your pleasure depends
on your wiring and your experiences. Some people like a lot of
adrenaline and the excitation of danger, others prefer a warm
glow in one of the energy centers.

What about physical pleasure?

Same principle. An excitation of energy someplace in
the body, or all over the body. A touch, a caress, sends a little
energy into the skin. You may process it as a local sensation,
or as something that activates a whole pattern in your body.
How often a warm caress brings a warm glow to our hearts!

We can control where the caress takes us. If we choose, we can melt our energy into it, inviting more of it. We can stiffen, and refuse it admittance, shutting off the energy flow. If we refuse admittance often enough, people learn not to touch us. If we project refusal, people won't think of touching us.

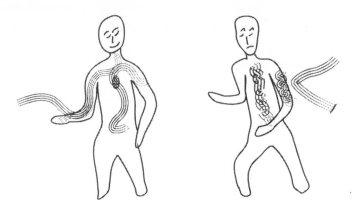

Let's see what the energy pattern is like.

Place your arm in a comfortable position, and caress it with your other hand. What does it feel like? Change the direction, the angle, the pressure, until your skin feels sensitized. Feel your arm with your hand, feel your hand with your arm.

As you begin your next caress, breathe in, and breathe down as you complete the caress. Your arm will relax, and the sensation will change a little.

Breathe in on your next caress, and as you breathe out, imagine the sensation running up your arm all the way to your head.

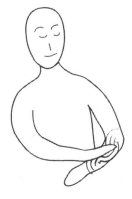 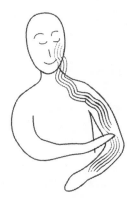

Explore this, seeing how you can connect the caress to the sensation and movement of your arm, shoulder, neck and head. Breathe in and breathe down, and see where it takes you.

You can consciously enhance the sensation by opening up an energy center.

Try another caress. Breathe in as you begin, and when you breathe out, open your heart energy to your arm. If it helps, imagine a line connecting your heart with your arm. How does it feel different? Does the motion feel warmer? Does your chest move now when you caress your arm?

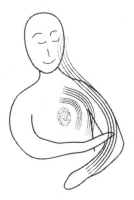

In earlier exercises, we connected different energy centers and parts of the body to see what it felt like. We were able to sense more, and feel more energy, by using our awareness. In the same way, we can enhance pleasure by using our awareness.

All it takes is paying attention to the stimulus, the energy, and opening to it so that it creates a heightening of sensation, of tension, followed by a release.

Breathe a small sigh. Feel how your chest expands and releases. Breathe a big sigh and let it run down your body into the ground. A very different feeling, isn't it?

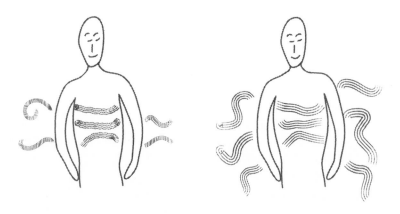

Doesn't pleasure just happen?

Yes, we are hard-wired to feel pleasure, because if pain is an irritation of our circuits, pleasure is a smoothing out. A little bit of pleasure soothes us, a lot of pleasure blows the circuits and releases a lot of tension.

Then why pay attention?

Pleasure smooths out our circuits, calms us, leaves us refreshed. But there is a pattern of diminishing returns. When does a pleasure stop giving the same satisfaction? Once you have smoothed out the circuits, what does repeating the pleasure accomplish?

As we evolve into more energy and more complexity, we need to find new ways of heightening and releasing our new patterns. That is exactly what we use our awareness for.

19 Neither pain nor pleasure

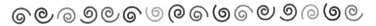

Pain hurts, pleasure feels good. What is neither one?

Many things. Good and evil, love and hatred, desire and rejection, open and closed. We seem to be surrounded by many boundaries, constantly trying to find our way through these choices.

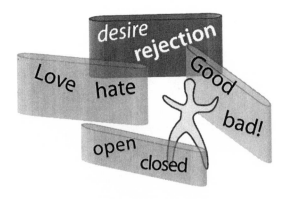

Aren't all these things more connected than separate?

Yes, they are. They are all patterns of energy flow, even dualities like love and hatred. Love is using the heart chakra to receive, process and send out energy. All the energy channels are open and sensitized. They pour energy into the open heart chakra. The flow is not linear or mechanical: all the channels are working together with the energy center in the heart as the main focus. The energy is greatly magnified if someone is sending heart energy back to you!

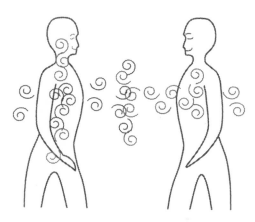

What, then, is hatred?

Hatred is closing off the heart chakra while still trying to funnel energy through it. The energy spins around the closed part, the hurt part, the part that needs to be protected. Closing off the whole chakra produces a cold, unemotional hatred. Closing off just a part can still use emotional frequencies and produces a "hot" hatred. Like a spinning hurricane, the results can be spectacular.

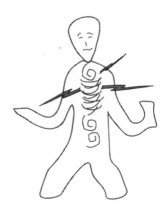

Love and hatred are both intense, dense with energy and sensation. The same patterns can also be run with less energy. Things we like but don't love. Experiences that leave us indifferent. A whole spectrum of possibilities in just one energy center!

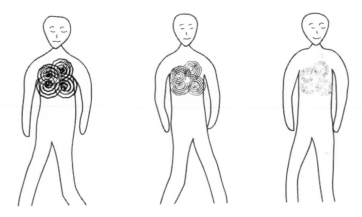

Add spectrums of possibilities for the other six energy centers, and all the possible combinations of those patterns, and we begin to see that duality is not really a very good model for describing the way we feel.

Pain, pleasure, love, hatred, desire, rejection are all patterns of energy that interact with each other, creating a stream more complex than any of its parts.

How do the patterns interact?

Think of a stained glass window you have seen. All the colors, the shapes. Light comes in from the back, is absorbed in different frequencies by different colors in the glass, and reaches your eyes in shapes and colors. You can look at different parts of the window: love and hatred, desire and rejection. They have their own stories, but they are all part of the greater pattern of the whole window. And the window is energy coming in, being absorbed, and being sent out in different frequencies and shapes.

We can think of the metal that holds the glass as our hard wiring, inherited from billions of years of evolution. Human aggressiveness, sociability, dominance patterns, mating patterns, tribal patterns form a structure that we all work with.

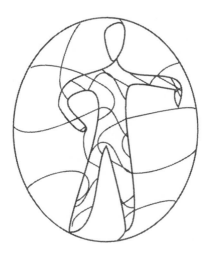

But the glass! The glass is heated and cooled; it changes color, shape, texture and clarity. It is red, blue, streaked or uniform, milky or clear. It is made of all the experiences you have had in your life, each contributing its own energy, its own color and qualities.

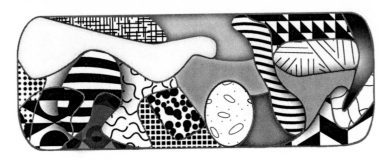

We change, though...

Yes, the glass is always changing. How marvelous! Not being fixed, we invent our own colors and shapes. But of course, we're not really talking about glass, we're talking about the textures and qualities of our life.

So how do we change the textures and qualities?

In much the same way as we experience a stained glass window. Seeing the light coming in, the light coming out. Noticing the structure, the shapes and colors. Focusing back and forth from the whole to the particular. Paying exquisite attention to everything.

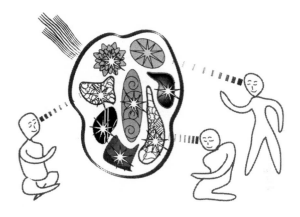

Exquisite attention…

When you feel pain, pay exquisite attention to the center of it, the edges of it, what it is telling you. When you feel pleasure, examine in your body what it feels like, where it peaks, where the tension releases, what the languid aftermath is like. Notice what you are thinking about and how your body is moving as you are thinking those thoughts. Tug on both mind and body to see what kind of tension is associated with those thoughts. Release some of the energy tied up in that pattern and see what happens.

We've been doing this, haven't we?

Yes. In our exercises we have been sharpening our awareness of our breath, our movement, our tension, our pain, and our pleasure. Sharpening our awareness of energy centers and different frequencies.

Once you learn to pay attention to what you are doing, you have the opportunity to pay exquisite attention to what you are doing.

How?

Slow down the movements, stretch out the moments. Breathe down, stretch your body, notice the pattern of sensation, be it tension, pain, pleasure. Notice the thoughts and emotions that come and go as you slowly move your body. Linger over each moment of awareness.

Switch your awareness from the movement of your body to your thoughts or emotions. As you notice them, move your body slowly and see what connections there are in the body to your mind.

Pay attention to the transitions. When you move from one position to another, slow it down, and notice each incremental change.

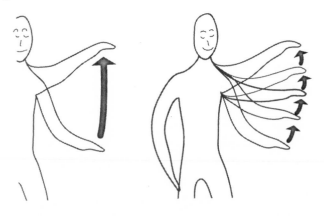

Sensations such as pain or pleasure, anger or fear or desire, tell us where energy densities are in the body and mind. When you are jumping between sensations, between densities, between points that you know well, you can whip through the energy channels to get there quicker. How quickly we can transform one pattern of feeling into another!

Where is the place that is neither pain nor pleasure? It is the connection between them, a place we usually rush through.

It is the place that tells us how pain and pleasure connect to each other in our own bodies.

As children we learned to connect the dots in simple drawings. As adults, seeing the whole picture is a matter of connecting the dots with exquisite attention, both the outline and the connections!

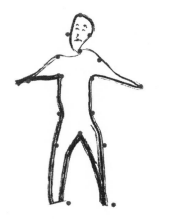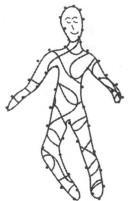

20 Inside-out, outside-in

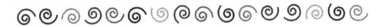

A new set of boundaries to explore!

Exactly. Like left and right, up and down, we can explore from the inside-out and the outside-in.

When we explored our knee with our head, we extended our awareness from the inside of our head to the outside of our knee. We worked back in the opposite direction, and then joined the two together. Let's explore that again.

Seat yourself comfortably. Breathe in, and breathe down, settling yourself.

Bring your head and knee together in a comfortable position. Breathe in and breathe down to relax.

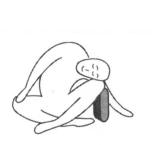
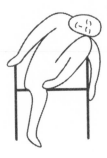

Feel your knee with your head. Breathe in, and breathe out from your head through your knee. Extend to the outside of knee, as if you were enfolding your knee with your head.

Move your awareness to your knee. Breathe in, and breathe out from your knee up and around your head.

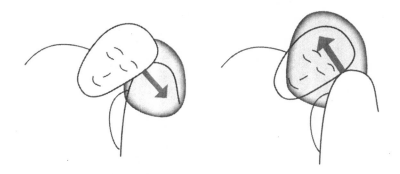

This is working inside-out, working from wherever our awareness is out to something else.

And outside-in?

It's like enfolding someone with a blanket to warm them. When you put a blanket around someone and hug them, you are placing yourself around their outside, and then bringing your energy into them from your arms, your chest, your head. Feels pretty good from both sides!

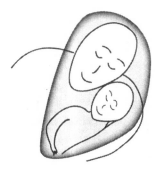

You can experience this yourself in your own body. Let's try a variation on our experience with the head and knee. Lie on your side with your knees drawn up together so that they are touching, one on top of the other.

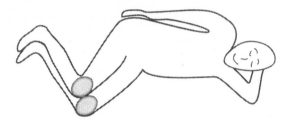

Breathe in, and breathe down, relaxing the body. Breathe in, and let your breath flow from the bottom knee up through the top knee. Breathe in, and let the top knee enfold the bottom one. Let them join together so that they have one outside boundary.

The knees are major joints in the body, and most of us carry tension in them. The sensation of letting them merge is quite relaxing and unmistakable!

Feel your joined knees as a single sensation. Feel around the edges of that sensation. When you can feel the whole boundary of your joined knees, breathe in. Breathe out from your joined knees to expand a little beyond them. Stay there.

Breathe in. When you breathe out, come back from the expanded boundary and feel your joined knees from the outside.

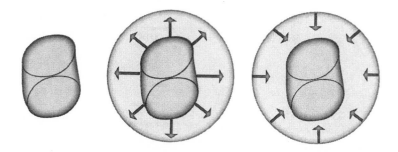

The sensation will be quite noticeable: your body position will shift a little, your breath will release, your knees will feel a little tingly. You'll know when you do it!

What is the difference between focusing inside-out or outside-in?

Not that much, actually. It's just the difference in where we place our awareness. There are lots of places in our bodies that have both an inside and an outside. Our shoulder joint, for example, is a ball and socket joint. The ball is held in the socket by connective tissue.

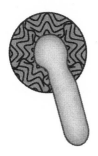

So we have an inside ball and an outside socket. Let's see what we can find.

Seat yourself comfortably, breathe in and breathe down. Feel for your right shoulder, imagining a ball of bone nestled in connective tissue. Put a little tension on it. Breathe in, and let the energy of your breath flow out in all directions from that ball.

This may take a few tries; we know our arm moves, but most of us don't pay close attention to the pieces. When you get it, there will be a feeling of warmth in the center of your shoulder joint.

When you have the sensation, breathe in and let your awareness jump a little outside the ball in all directions. Stabilize this new outer boundary. Breathe in, and breathe back into the center of the ball.

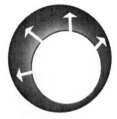 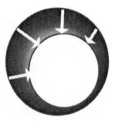

Play with your breathing and the sensation. Moving out from the ball produces warmth in the center of the shoulder. Moving in from the socket tends to relax the whole joint.

Try it with your other shoulder. Try it with your hip joints, which are constructed similarly. The tension is greater in the hip joint, and the release will feel greater, as well.

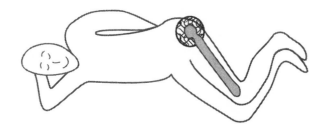

Try relaxing all four joints at the same time, both shoulders and both hips. It is a delicious sensation to relax all of them at once!

We're releasing energy in the joints from inside and outside...

Yes. It's just another direction, like left and right, up and down, front and back. But it is a direction that allows us to venture further afield, to inside and outside of *us*.

What we did with our knees, we can do with our bodies and the ground. Sit comfortably cross-legged on the ground. Breathe in, and breathe down, settling your self.

Feel how your weight sits on the ground, notice the angle of your legs and whether they are tense or relaxed. Breathe in, and breathe down, relaxing everything. Feel the triangle of your legs and pelvis. Let them join together in one large boundary.

Breathe in, and breathe down into the ground from the triangle, as far as you can. Stay there a moment and feel the new boundary.

Breathe in at the new boundary. Breath out from the boundary back up to your lower body.

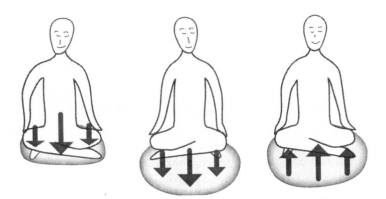

This is another unmistakable sensation, much the same as breathing from the shoulder or hip socket into the ball of the joint.

Although looking at things from inside and outside is less common to us than left or right, top or bottom, it is not at all outside our experience. When we taste good food, there is a moment when it tastes so good we become the flavor. And with a pleasantly full stomach, are we the stomach holding the food, or the food filling the stomach?

What we think of as inside and outside is malleable. When we make love, there is often a moment when we are not sure which arms and legs belong to us, and which belong to the other person. What we define as inside and outside changes from moment to moment.

So we can move the boundaries?

As we like, as often as we like. All we have to do is adjust our attention. When you shower, let the water run onto your head or neck a moment. Feel the drops hitting your skin. Move your attention outward to where the skin and drops meet, where the skin is dancing with the drops.

Move it outward once more, into the water that is falling onto your skin. With practice, you can extend your attention all the way up and down the stream of water.

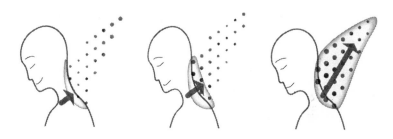

As you open to the water, think of how much fun it was as a child to play in the rain!

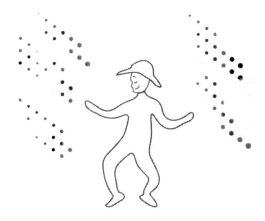

21 Advanced wiring

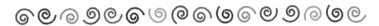

Advanced?

Well, more advanced than we've discussed so far! After you start exploring the wiring of the body, there are many things to discover.

For example, the front of your body and the back of your body are different energy channels. The front is a receiver and sender of energy. The back is too, but we rarely use it. Instead, we keep it closed for protection.

Have you ever seen a child concentrate? They will stare at a pebble in the sand with all of their being. Their whole body will focus, everything facing one direction.

Our senses are stronger to the front because they are all lined up to work together: ears, face, throat, heart, and pelvis. The front is where we spend the most time, taking in and sending out energy.

We put a face on things, face forward, face the music, get things off our chest. We put the best face on things and never turn our back to the audience.

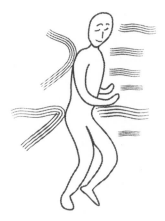

Our back is where things bounce off us. We back up, turn our backs, get things off our back or behind us. People from the backwoods are backwards.

So the front is forward and the back is, well... back.

Only if we look at it from the front! Let's open each chakra from both the front and the back and see what perspectives we find.

Seat yourself comfortably, breathe in, and breathe down, relaxing.

Breathe in, and breathe out through the front of the heart past your skin into the space in front of you. Breathe in, and breathe out through the back of the heart into the space behind you. Feels different the second time, doesn't it? Bigger, broader.

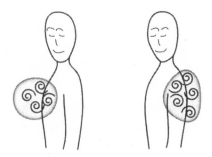

Explore opening different chakras, opening the front and back. Does it feel different if you open the back up first? Opening the back may be a little more work than opening the front, because we tend to keep the backs of the chakras closed most of the time.

Open them one at a time. See how many you can be aware of at the same time.

At the same time?

People often lead with one energy center. With a child you might lead from the heart, with a friend you might lead from the mind, and with a lover you might at times lead from the pelvis.

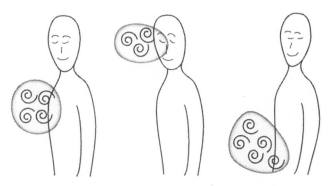

When we meet somebody we are interested in, we may use first mind, then heart, then pelvis to see what all the possibilities are.

Sometimes we lead with one chakra to hide the others. Have you ever had a conversation with someone who nervously just kept talking? The talking is real, but it also is to distract you from noticing the rest of their energy.

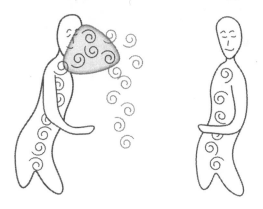

We use combinations, too. Evolving different kinds of patterns throughout our lives.

What kind of patterns?

There are many patterns. One example is mind and throat, noticeable when someone talks a lot and spins out ideas endlessly. They can sound rather breathless at times.

Another pattern is throat and heart, all words and emotions. Another is one we associate with sexual magnetism, using the second and breath chakras. The energy in the breath chakra helps propel the sexual energy outward to others, and together they have more energy than the second chakra by itself.

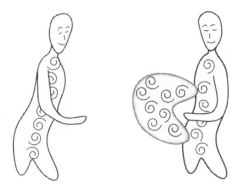

Sometimes the energy pattern isn't based in the chakras. For example, humans are extravagantly equipped with wiring for sensation between the second and breath chakras. An area in which the loudest organ is the stomach. It's an easy place for humans to put their attention.

We pay attention to our stomachs when we are hungry or nervous or upset. We relax when our stomachs relax. Think how nice a warm, full stomach feels!

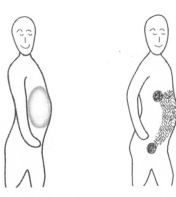

The area between the second and breath chakras has good wiring. Wiring necessary for survival. For knowing when to get food, to tell what foods are good for you. For monitoring sickness and health. We can rely on this so much that we can lead with our stomachs, with everything else trailing behind!

Hey, I might resemble that!

We all do at times! The channels between the second and breath chakras are an important part of our lives. Place energy and awareness into them. Just don't expect that they can be a substitute for the stronger energy channels in the chakras.

For clear perception, it's more useful to use the main energy channels. We need only to open up the chakras and connect them.

We've already opened each one...

And now we connect the dots. Go ahead and open all your chakras again, one at a time, by breathing out from the front and back of each chakra.

Center your awareness in your head, and draw a line with your mind to your heart. You'll feel the connection instantly when it happens.

The line we've drawn is a straight line, so let's bring the throat chakra into the line. Just bring the energy of the throat center forward until it touches the line between the mind and the heart. It will snap into place.

Extend the line downward, one chakra at a time, into the ground. This is your front channel. Rest a moment and enjoy it!

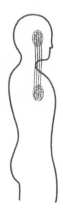 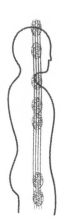 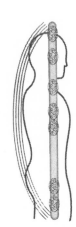

Now for the back channel. Imagine the front channel as a bowstring, with the bow itself curving just outside your back. The bowstring connects to the bow at the top and bottom.

Breathe in, and breathe out through the back of your heart towards the bow. When you lock in the heart energy to the bow, the energy will travel from the center to the ends of the bow.

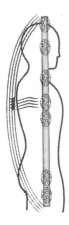 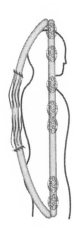

Wow. Front and back channels.

Explore the difference in how they feel. Move your body into different positions, feeling the tension in the front, and the tension in the back. Keep the sense of the bow and the bowstring as you move, feeling how it changes shape with each movement.

As you find different patterns of tension, try releasing them. Breathe in, and breathe down, releasing tension on the bowstring. And releasing tension on the bow, as well!

Now that we have a good sense of where the two channels are, let's explore further by running energy through the front and back. Breathe in with your pelvis, widening your hips as you breathe in. Breathe out and up through the bowstring, your front channel.

Breathe in, and breathe up through the bow, your back channel. Explore the channels, breathing in from the bottom or the top, running up or down the front or back.

Try everything you can think of!

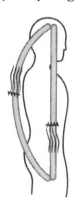 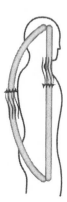 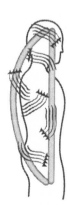

We use the front and back channels all the time, often without paying much attention. When we rise up to confront someone, we breathe up through the front, using the energy to

stiffen all the muscles in the front, appear taller, and increase
the front energy to face someone.

When we shrink away, we breathe down the back,
grounding our energy, curving our back and becoming smaller,
less confronting.

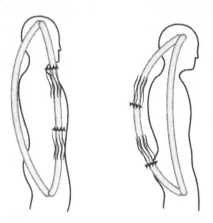

These are two examples of how we use our channels
automatically. Let's try exploring them consciously.

Stay with your awareness of your front and back channels.
Think of different people you know, different situations you
encounter at home, work, or in town. Notice how the channels
change with each thought. They may change slightly or
dramatically. They may charge up or relax down.

The front and back channels are always firing like clouds
chasing each other across a sky. Changing every moment.
Heating up, cooling down. Charging the rest of the circuits in
complex patterns.

Complex patterns?

Very complex. What we've described so far as the front
channel is actually a combination of two channels, one in

front of the other. The more forward channel reflects the expanding nature of the universe. Let's call this the shiva channel. The deeper one reflects the encompassing nature of the universe. Let's call this the shakti channel. Together, they offer an extraordinary number of possibilities.

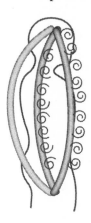

You said earlier that Shakti was the feminine principle of the universe.

It is often described that way, just as Shiva is described as the male principle. Since humans themselves are male and female, we describe many things that way! In some human languages, everything is either male or female.

The universe, however, is prior to male and female, just as asexual reproduction came earlier in evolution than sexual reproduction.

Where do these principles came from?

As far as we know, the universe was born 13.7 billion years ago. From the moment of the Big Bang, it has been expanding, pushing outward in all directions. It has also been continuously encompassing its growing self as it expands. If there is a primal duality in the universe that duality would be inside and outside, expanding and encompassing. If it is hard-wired into the universe, it is hard-wired into us!

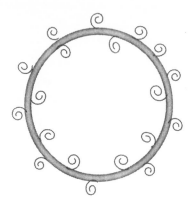

Hard-wired? How?

Both channels run through the chakras, but very differently. The shiva channel is out front. The energy from it is always pushing forward. The easiest way to find the shiva channel is to lean forward, so that you can draw a straight line from your base chakra to your head. When you connect them, breathe up the front. It will feel like a rubber band!

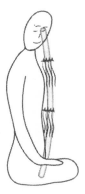

The shakti channel lies deeper. Straighten your body so that your head is back. Feel for the four tension points of the circuit. Two are in the creases of the hips, two are in the crease of the shoulder below the collarbone. Feel for all four, and breathe up through all of them.

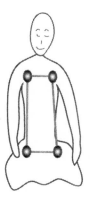 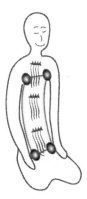

Where the shiva circuit felt like a straight line, the shakti circuit feels more like a half-cylinder or cup. It feels much like the back channel, but if you open up your back, you will certainly feel the difference!

So everyone has both shiva and shakti channels?

Yes. Some people use more shiva energy, some use more
shakti. If you think of shiva as pushing boundaries and shakti
as nurturing, you see immediately that everyone has some
combination of both. It's a bell curve with most people in the
middle and some people much more one than the other.

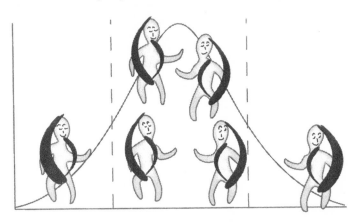

Does male and female matter?

Yes, though not as much as you might think. The physical
difference between men and women promotes shiva in men,
shakti in women. Men have an easier time finding the shiva
channel, women an easier time finding the shakti channel.

See if you can find both channels, and the back channel,
in different positions. Breath down in each position to take the
tension out of the channels.

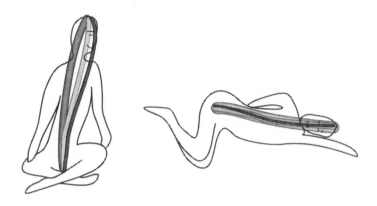

As you work with them, do they begin to vibrate or warm up? Good. Then we discuss what happens when they get *hot!*

22 Hot wiring

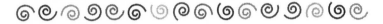

What is hot wiring?

Like a toaster, circuits get warm. Then they glow. At a certain point, the wiring catches fire.

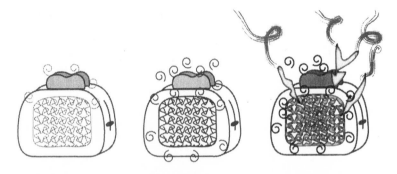

Human wiring is much the same. When children run around playing there is an exuberance about them that is endearing. They glow with excitement and pleasure.

At some point they lose control of the energy, the circuits keep firing, and the energy starts to spike erratically. They get irritated, angry, or cry uncontrollably. What parent has not, at some point, apologetically explained that their child is over-stimulated?

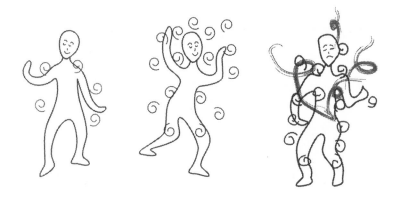

Is it physical or energetic?

From both perspectives, the energy heats up the circuit, the circuit starts glowing, the circuit combusts.

Combustible circuits are part of our every-day experience. The buildup and explosion of energy is hard-wired into us, and is the basic pattern of that most mysterious activity, sex.

Sex is hot wiring and an explosion of energy?

Sex heats up the wires. The explosion is orgasm. We can think of them together as a heating and explosion of the second chakra.

Other chakras can heat up and explode, too. The crown chakra can explode in meditation, the mind chakra can explode with insight, the heart chakra can explode with love, the base chakra can explode with fear.

Each of these explosions flood the entire body with frequencies of energy. The frequencies of the second chakra, which we call desire and passion, are great energizers both of our lives and of our cultures.

Chakras do not exist in isolation. They are part of all
the wiring in the body. The second chakra has a wealth of
connections to the circuits in the pelvis.

We already know that the pelvis is a crossroads, anchoring
both the legs and the upper body. We've breathed down
through the pelvis to release tension throughout our whole
body. We have seen that the pelvis itself is not a solid
structure, but has its own patterns of tension.

We flexed our pelvis in different directions...

Yes. That swirls things around nicely. Let's look more
closely at what gets swirled around. To begin with, there is the
connection between the first and second chakras.

When we talked earlier about opening the first and second
chakras, we mentioned making space between them. The
first chakra is below the pubic bone in the triangle between
the bottom of the pubic bone and the sit bones. The closest
physical location is the perineum, a patch of smooth skin in
front of the anus.

The second chakra is located a little above and behind the
top of the pubic bone. When the pelvis is under tension, the
two are drawn closer together.

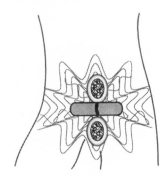

Take a moment to separate them. Sit in a comfortable position. Bring your awareness to your pubic bone. Expand it as you breathe in. Breathe down from the pubic bone, dropping your sit-bones into the ground.

Breathe in again, expanding the pubic bone. Breathe up from the pubic bone, raising your chest and stretching your abdomen.

Breathe in, and breathe both down and up.

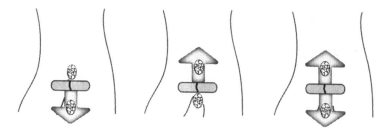

That's a strong sensation!

There is a lot of tension in the pubic bone. It is the front pivot point of the two large pelvic bones of the pelvis. The back pivot point is the dense connections between the sacrum and the pelvic bones, the sacroiliac joint.

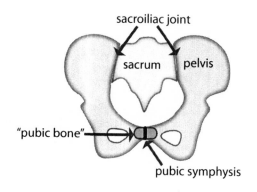

The pubic bone is actually two separate bones, the front pieces of the pelvic bones. It is held together by a dense weaving of connective tissue called the pubic symphysis. The symphysis is considered a slightly moveable joint, meaning it is held very tightly. Tightly enough so that women in childbirth secrete hormones to help it loosen.

We pay a lot of attention to the pubic bone, though rarely with awareness. Children instinctively press on their pubic bone when under stress, until they are taught not to do so.

We pay the most attention to the pubic bone in adolescence. It aches as it grows and tightens to its adult size, shape, weight and tension. It aches under stress, too.

It aches for adults, as well, though we often may ignore it. It aches with tension, and aches with relief. It tightens for danger and for sex; it relaxes when tension is released.

Let's see if we can better identify that tension.

Lie on your back with a pillow or block underneath your sacrum, or on the edge of a bed. Breathe in and breathe down to relax.

Feel the triangle formed by the two outside points of your pelvis and the center of your pubic bone, the symphysis.

Breathe in, and breathe up through the symphysis. As you release tension, your pelvis will expand from the center and your body will relax.

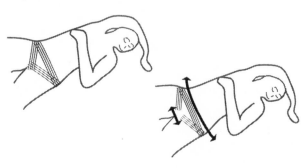

Opening the symphysis can produce a lot of sensation and energy on its own. But this is also where the genitals attach. Add the exquisite sensitivity and response of the genitals to the energy locked in the pubic bone and pubic symphysis, and you begin to see why sexual excitement and release looms so large in human lives and culture.

The tension on the pubic bone and pubic symphysis varies among humans, particularly between males and females.

In what way?

Even a casual look at the male and female pelvis shows a distinct difference in structure. Anthropologists often use the difference to identify the sex of human fossils.

The male pelvis is taller and heavier. The larger size allows for stronger muscle attachments and more physical power. The symphysis is longer, deeper, and tighter.

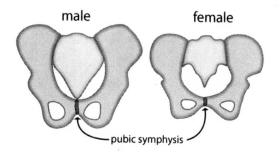

In males the symphysis is also more forward, with more of a straight line to the head. Increased size, weight, tension, and forward position accentuates the forward shiva channel in men.

When the forward shiva channel tightens, so does the front of the body, creating a more direct line between the brain and the symphysis. This comes in handy when visuals of danger create a need to tighten the base chakra for protection and change the center of balance to poise for fight or flight.

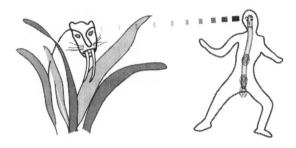

The stronger shiva channel in men means that male energy is more forward. This makes sense in terms of sexual reproduction. In mammals, the male moves DNA from his body forward to the female, who receives it.

It also makes evolutionary sense, since men tended to focus forward on hunting animals in the landscape. Women traditionally focused more on scanning the landscape for edibles, a more receptive activity than hunting.

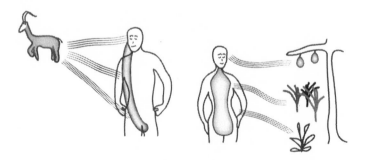

The stronger shiva channel in men ties their genitals more directly to the brain. It's why men are much more affected by visuals such as pornography. It's why every human culture jokes about a man's brain being in his genitals.

Remember the bell curve, though. It's a range of variation. Variation in male pelvises, female pelvises, male and female body types. Variation in personal experience that create different patterns of tension in the symphysis and pelvis.

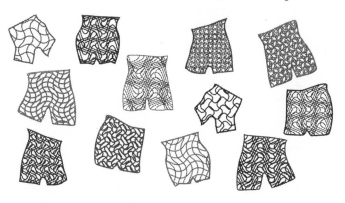

Everybody feels the shiva channel differently, uses it differently.

And the shakti channel?

The shakti channel lies deeper in the pelvis and in the body. It's broader than the shiva channel. The shiva channel feels more electric, the shakti channel feels more sinuous. The shiva channel goes up the front, the shakti channel spreads throughout the body.

Do we use both then?

We should! And the back channel, as well. But before we can see how, we need to explore the energy in the pelvis a little further.

The entire pelvis is an energy circuit. Moving the pelvis loosens connections and releases energy to warm the channels. Sports and dance are two examples of how the pelvis warms and throws off energy that can feel very much like erotic energy.

We can how see the energy moves in the pelvis by expanding the pelvis with the in-breath and following the movement of the out-breath.

Seat yourself comfortably, breathe in, and breathe down into the ground.

Breathe in, expanding the circle of your hips to the side. Notice the tension on the pubic symphysis and sacrum. Breath out and let the pelvis fall back in. Breathe a couple times, feeling for the way the circle moves.

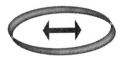 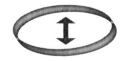 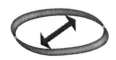

Change the direction. Try expanding front and back to breathe in. Try diagonals.

When you have a sense of the whole pelvis, expand the whole circle on the in-breath. Move your awareness around the circle with the out-breath, clockwise and counter-clockwise. Try both directions at once, inside and outside!

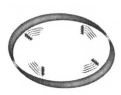 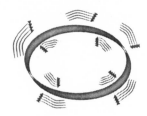

Try a different position. Lay back and twist your body. Feel for the circle of the pelvis with its joints in front and back. Breathe with your pelvis in the new position. Loosening the pelvis is like loosening any other part of the body: energy used for binding things tightly is released to circulate in the energy system.

Back channel, shakti channel, shiva channel, and pelvis. All we need is the ignition switch: our erogenous zones.

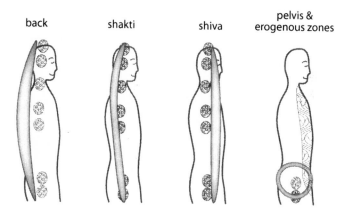

Erogenous zones are the ignition?

Yes. Erogenous zones are patterns of sensitivity. They are the heat that warms the circuits. When we become aroused, the body rushes blood to them, warming them, stimulating them, and adding extra energy.

Every human has a unique pattern of sensitivity. Overlaid on the hard-wired physical responses are cultural patterns of how you "should" feel your body. Added to those are the patterns evolved from our past experience and response.

Still, erogenous patterns fall along a bell curve, with most people sharing similar patterns of sensitivity, but with many humans feeling something quite different.

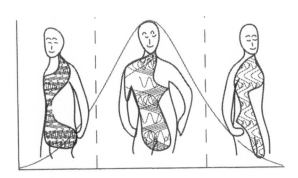

The erogenous zones warm up quickly and pulse energy through the body. The mind focuses on the sensation, amplifying it. The pelvis warms and begins to move. The movement further stimulates the erogenous zones. The energy builds on itself until the system hits a tipping point, a butterfly point.

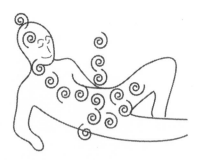

And then the explosion?

That would be nice! But it doesn't always work that way. The wiring is more complicated than that.

If you don't connect the energy to the main channels, the sparks fizzle before they explode into fireworks.

23 How to explode fireworks

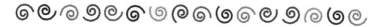

Okay, how do we explode fireworks?

With passion, of course! And energy in the five circuits.

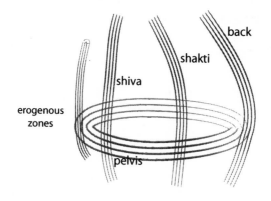

These circuits combine in many different ways, and each circuit is pulsing with energy from moment to moment. Not just during sex, but all the time.

As a circuit warms, the energy builds, until the circuit explodes, firing energy in all directions. On a physical level, it can be described as the build-up and release of tension.

In thermodynamic terms, a circuit builds energy until the existing pattern cannot hold it any longer and encounters a butterfly point. The system can either evolve to an expanded level of energy, or release the energy. Or both. The word we usually use for the release during sex is *orgasm*.

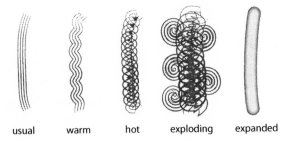

usual   warm   hot   exploding   expanded

After the energy is released, the circuit, still hot and expanded, settles into a calm glow. If the circuit is low-energy, then the circuit can only expand a little. The extra energy is simply released, and there is very little glow. If the circuit has a lot of energy, there is potential for both releasing a lot of energy and a much bigger glow.

Energy in a circuit can be released all at once or a bit at a time. Sometimes, if the circuit becomes over-stimulated, the energy will simply drain away into the physical body. The sparks fizzle.

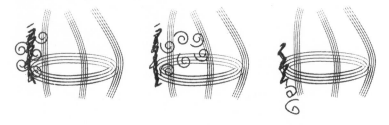

Humans are designed to have sex. The basic hard-wiring works with or without awareness. Just the explosion of the erogenous circuit of a male into a female is enough for procreation. Most humans, though, would consider this to be of limited satisfaction. With repetition, it can actually become boring.

It is much more satisfying to involve as many channels as we can, enhancing the energy and sensitivity. The more energy we raise in the channels, the more they evolve to accommodate increased energy. Not just for sex, for everything.

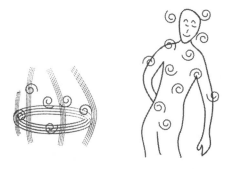

How do we raise energy?

It's instinctual to swirl together the physical pleasure, the tension, the desire of the second chakra, and the heart energy of the heart chakra until it fountains over. It is all too true, though, that cultural and individual patterns can get in the way. That's where awareness comes in.

In our exercises we've gotten a lot of experience with building and releasing tension in our bodies. How much tension is enough? How much is too much? How much release occurs? Where does it go?

The answers vary with every person and every flowing moment, but the five circuits provide the wiring.

The erogenous circuit has great sensitivity but can handle less energy than the other circuits. It is very good at transferring energy to the shiva and shakti channels, and very good at stimulating the pelvis into motion.

The pelvis contains a great deal of energy, both because of its own wiring and because the first and second chakras are there. It is from the second chakra that the energy moves up the shiva and shakti channels.

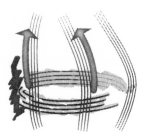

What we describe as an orgasm is usually the release of either the shiva channel or the shakti channel. A shiva channel release is more forward and feels like a lightning bolt; the electric energy runs from the front of the pelvis up through the head. Men tend to have a stronger shiva channel, use it more often, rely on it more. Men generally find the shiva channel release more satisfying than do women.

A shakti channel release feels more like an earthquake! The energy release lies deeper in the pelvis, and travels up the broader shakti channel through the body and to either side of the head.

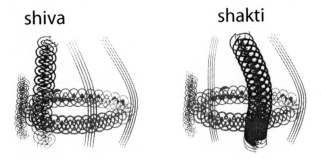

shiva   shakti

Do people have either a shiva or a shakti release?

All humans have both channels, though they may rely almost exclusively on one. The release of one channel will affect the others to some extent.

Both channels can release at the same time for spectacular fireworks. This often happens spontaneously when both get hot enough to combust.

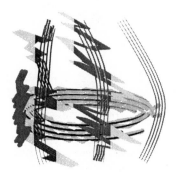

What about the back channel?

If the release of the shiva/shakti channels is fireworks, the back channel feels like the whole sky. Let's explore the back channel with a breath exercise. We'll connect through the back of each chakra.

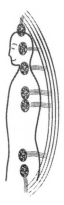

Sit comfortably, breathe in, and breathe down. Notice the end of the breath and pause. Breathe in and breathe down, and when you reach the pause, send the energy down as through dropping a weight on a string. Where the weight ends up is *down*. Breathe a couple times to anchor your sense of where *down* is in your body.

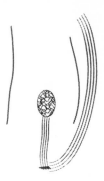 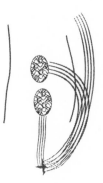

Now for the second chakra. Breathe in, and breathe out through the back of the pelvis. Follow your breath, and curve down around your back and find *down*. You will definitely feel the connection when you make it!

Hold the connection if you can, but don't worry about it. Open the back-door of the other chakras. Open as many as you can at the same time. After a few tries, you will be able to connect the whole line of the back channel.

Wow, my back feels bigger!

The sensation feels like a flower opening, or a door expanding. With a little practice, you can open your back channel quite easily, simply by breathing out the sides of your back.

The back channel can also warm and open spontaneously when all five circuits release in orgasm. All the circuits will release at the same time if the butterfly point, the tipping point of the orgasm, is at the nexus of all five energy channels.

The locus, which some have tried to identify in a physical location called the *G-Spot*, is not a constant physical place. Let's call it the *U-Spot*.

The U-Spot moves from moment to moment as the pelvis moves and the energy moves. You can try and chase it, but it is much easier to find if you first heat all the channels and then look for where they connect.

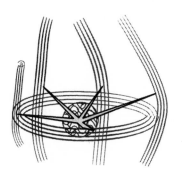 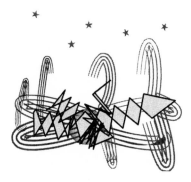

If you can release all five channels at the same time, you get the fireworks, the earthquake, and the whole night sky.

That's it, then!

There's so much more to explore! There are many different patterns of warming and exploding in our body. Many different patterns of awareness.

With awareness we can make new patterns at every moment. We can run different amounts of energy in each circuit, and swirl the energy from circuit to circuit.

With awareness...

How much attention do we pay to what we are doing? How much energy do we divert into protection or fear or shame, or maintaining our personality while our body is trying to loosen up?

What is our intent?

Are we looking to release excess energy? Do we crave human contact and pleasure? Do we feel obligated? Are we trying to raise our energy state and awareness? Are we tuned to another human and want to merge with them?

Each different intent opens and closes different circuits. The more circuits we open with our awareness, the greater the fireworks.

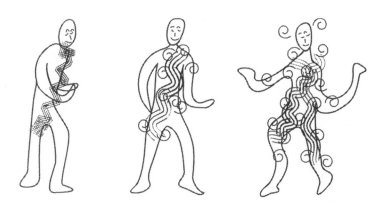

How DO we get fireworks?

By deliberately connecting the channels instead of just hoping for it. Move energy into the forward shiva channel. Move energy through the deeper shakti channel. Energize the pelvis. Keep the energy moving to get all of the channels hot.

Breathe in, and open the back channel. Drive the energy from the erogenous zones down into the sacrum.

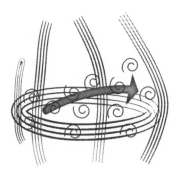

With a partner, connect the two second chakras. Connect the shiva channels, the shakti channels.

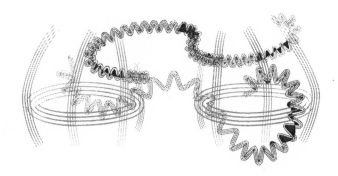

Work your attention back and forth from channel to channel, looking up and down for the exquisite points of tension and release.

Slow your breath down, especially when a release beckons. Look for the moment between two breaths, two movements. Savor the sensation. Breathe from the exploding channels into the back channels. Look to explode all the channels at the same time.

This may not happen the first time you try it. But it will happen if you want it, because the universe has given you the wiring!

What about techniques?

There is no technique in the world that is as effective as paying exquisite attention to your energy. Learning to use all your channels is making love with your whole body. This cannot be taught; you must explore your own path to more awareness.

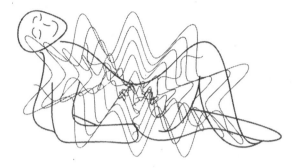

And there is no technique for opening your back channel and connecting to the universe. There is only the doing of it. And the exploring of what you discover in an expanded state.

24 Flowing passion, flowing play

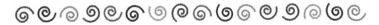

Are they related?

Passion and play are two ways we move through the universe. So much a part of our lives that it is very hard to step back and really look at them. Think of all the word associations we have!

There are burning passions, and long-simmering ones. Men are driven by their passions, but somehow women are more passionate. We speak of passions of the moment, crimes of passion, someone being in the throes of passion. People can be strong with passion, and made weak by passion.

Play is more elusive, more tenuous. As children we play at being adults. Serious adults are encouraged to play more, and playful adults are chastised for playing too much. We play roles, games, politics, and instruments. We are not supposed to play with our food.

We think of children as mostly playful, but they are also passionate about things. When adults throw themselves into games, we say they have a "passion for the game." Sex can be playful or passionate or both. So can art and music and dance.

How can we use the same words for so many things?

Different intensities?

Yes. Different frequencies, as well, since passion feels deeper than play. Passion and play both are forms of desire, a word we use to refer to the energy coming through the second chakra. Passion is the more intense form of desire; the stronger, deeper, more directed flow.

What do you have a passion for? Objects? Activities? People? How do you feel when you are feeling passionate?

Some people live for the passionate moments in their lives, or mourn the passionate moments left behind. It is when they feel the most alive, the most energetic. It is when the energy in the second chakra is most flowing.

Play is lighter in energy, but still flowing. It is more diffuse, more lyrical. Play is in and out, back and forth; it is of the moment.

Passion is a directed flow of energy; play is energy flowing for the pleasure of it.

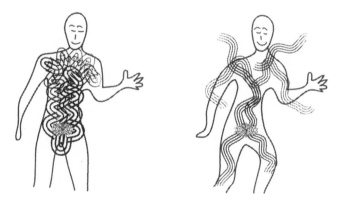

Humans of all ages have second chakra energy available for patterns of passion and play. Most children are good at play, because they are less governed by rules that channel their energy. They flow where their energy takes them. Adolescents are good at play, too. With the development of more channels at puberty they also become passionate about everything.

In some ways, desire is clearer for adolescents than for adults, because it is everywhere. For adults, desire has many more patterns to navigate, both individual and cultural. Often, desire is forced into defined patterns that are culturally acceptable.

Desire is so much a part of our energy flow that we often only notice it when it is frustrated!

What happens then?

Many things can happen. Sometimes we bring all our energy to bear on the object of our desire until we get it. This is usually unsatisfactory, since it is the intensity of the passion we crave, not the object. Sometimes we hold the desire inside ourselves and connect to it a whole pattern of thoughts, emotions and physical responses. Sometimes we let our desire flow freely into other directions.

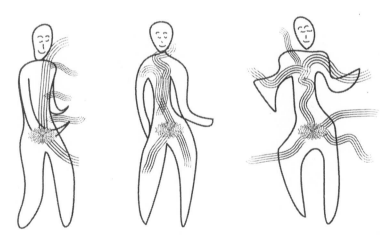

Think about your own or anyone else's life, and you can readily see how desire finds outlets, creates new patterns. We do this naturally. We do not always do it with awareness.

What things prompt us to feel desire? To be passionate? To be playful? How do we interact with our own desire? Our own energy?

Do we direct the energy or are we the energy itself? Or as the Irish poet William Butler Yeats asked, "How can you tell the dancer from the dance?"

Do you have an answer?

They are the same...

They often are. Opening to the flow of the dance, to the flow of desire, is ecstatic, radiant, joyful. It is a state connected to the flow of the universe. Connected to the passion and play of the universe itself.

How extraordinary, then, that there is also the interplay of the dancer and the dance. An interplay of awareness and energy we can explore in *Tandava*, the Tantric yoga dance.

Tandava...

Tandava has several traditional forms. Slower forms explore more of the awareness, faster forms are more focused on ecstatic energy. Let's first explore a slow form, similar to one taught by Daniel Odier, a dance of breath and exquisite attention to slow movements. We can call it every-breath Tandava.

Tandava is very simple, being just breath, awareness and movement, but not so easy to do. And not so easy to describe! It is done seated, standing or moving in space. Seated is easier and a good way to begin; there are fewer limbs to keep track of!

In Tandava, we focus first on the in-breath, and then watch how the energy moves as we breathe out. Then we notice the pause before the next in-breath. Let's try this.

Seat yourself comfortably, breathe in, and breathe down.
On the next breath down, drop a weight from your pelvis
down below the floor. Let it hang there a moment before
breathing in again.

Try this a few times, gradually increasing the "hang time."
This moment of stillness is a moment of full awareness, a
moment in which you are not using energy for anything else.

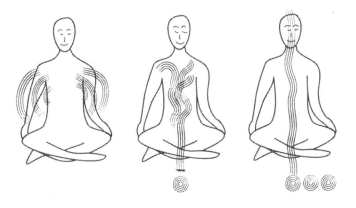

Now that we've clearly marked the pause after the out-
breath, we can reverse the flow of breath and let the energy go
through our body rather than grounding it.

For Tandava we will breathe from the pelvis. Expand your
hips as you breathe in. As your hips relax back inward, let the
breath flow up through your body to move your arms. When
you pause the breath, pause the movement, as well.

The sequence is breathe, move, pause... breathe, move,
pause.

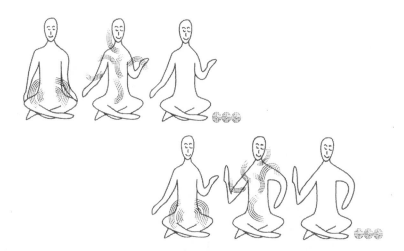

The pause at the end of the movement prevents your body from moving in pre-programmed patterns. Each new breath produces a different, unique movement.

Let your hands move of their own accord. Watch how they move. Let them move independently of each other. They will surprise you!

If you become tense from concentration, breathe down to relax before going back to your in-breath. Take a normal breath once in a while.

As you grow more comfortable with your breath and movement, begin to let your head move. When you are comfortable with the head movement, let your spine join the movement.

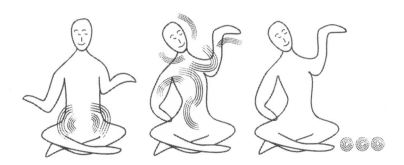

It is a great temptation to focus on the movement. It is easier. Your movements will speed up and become stronger, the breath used simply to push the movement.

When this happens, return to the in-breath from the pelvis and the energy running up through the body. Return to the pause after the movement.

This is hard!

Yes! You are tracking your in-breath, the energy movement in your body, and the way the body moves with the energy. You are paying attention to the separate movements of your breath, hands, head and spine while maintaining your awareness of all the transitions. Rest whenever when you get tired!

What are other forms of Tandava like?

Lots of fun! Especially with music. Dancing-hands Tandava focuses on the interaction of your hands and your awareness. The music should be rhythmic but not too repetitive.

Seat yourself comfortably with your hands held in front of you. Breathe in, and breathe down to relax.

Let your hands begin to dance to the music. Let them move of their own accord. Watch them flow around each other.

Let your awareness flow into the space between your hands. Let the dance become three-sided.

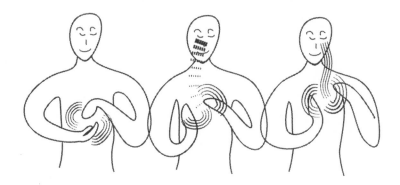

Keep your awareness with your hands as you dance with them. Focus on the left hand, the right hand, the space between them.

Try it standing, moving, dancing, spinning! Bring your feet into the dance, the oval of your pelvis, the circles of your chest and head. Focus on different chakras as you dance, seeing how changing the chakra changes the movements.

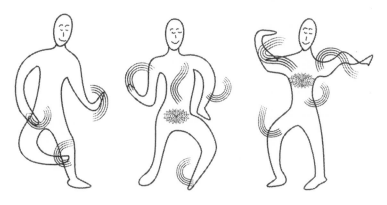

Whenever you begin to dance without awareness, bring
your attention back to your hands.

Play with all the elements, explore them any way you
will. For a minute, a few minutes, or an hour. Indoors
and outdoors, with music or without. You can make the
movements subtle enough to Tandava while standing in line
at a store. With everyone else moving from boredom and
impatience, no one will notice your Tandava until you smile!

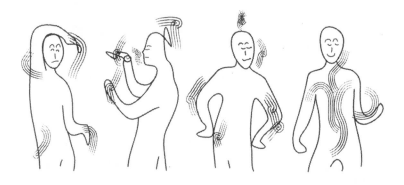

Tandava, Tandava, Tandava... and see for yourself how the
dancer and the dance are joined.

25 Clearing static

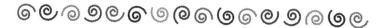

Static?

We're accustomed to thinking of static as electricity. Shuffle your feet on a carpet and touch a doorknob. Touch the ball of electricity in the museum and watch your hair stand on end!

Static is also the crackling noise we hear on the radio when the signal isn't clear. Or the flurry of energy we get from someone who doesn't like our suggestion.

Static is the tension and flyaway energy that surrounds us at the end of the day when we have dealt with too many things, too many ideas, too many people!

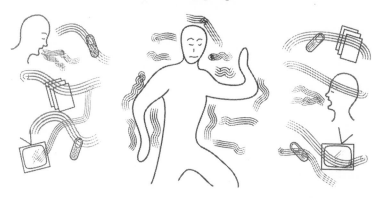

It is why we reach every day for our own end-of-day ritual: a drink, a cup of tea, a bath, a workout, family time. We sigh, we relax, we release the static energy.

We release the static...

Instinctively, yes. Static irritates us and produces tension. It fogs our vision, our senses. We act to reduce it to see and feel better.

When someone comes to us nervous or in a panic, throwing energy all around us, what do we do? Our first instinct is to put up our hands to keep it from reaching us. We then move our hands downward, grounding as much of it as we can. That helps clears the way for communication.

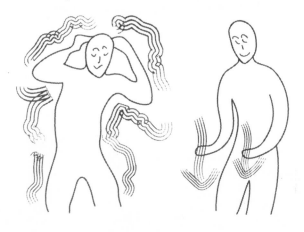

Actually, we do the same thing with ourselves when we feel the need to calm down!

Some people keep up a continuous flow of static, for many reasons. They may be keeping their energy so tense that they have to constantly shed the excess tension. They might project the static as a smokescreen that keeps other people away. Static keeps our awareness distracted. Too distracted to spare much energy for listening to the universe.

Static is part of life. Especially modern life. For centuries, mystics have lived on mountains, and in secluded places. They avoided the static of city and village life to get clarity, to get a clearer channel to the universe.

We live today in a fast-paced world filled with images, ideas and change. The Internet brings us energy/information from all over the world, wiring our minds to many other humans.

We know mind static very well! So let's start there.

Seat yourself comfortably. Breathe in, and breathe down. Breathing down helps clear the static from the base chakra.

Clearing static is much like breathing out through the front and back of a chakra. Where we focused earlier on the breath, now we will focus on the edge of the breath.

If it helps, think of your head as a balloon. As it expands it fills with air. As it releases air it falls back to the center.

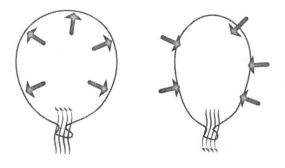

Breathe in, expanding your head as though it were your lungs. Release. Play with this until the whole balloon is expanding and contracting.

Breathe in and expand. Feel the sides of the balloon and hold the tension a moment. Release your breath outward, expanding the balloon further. When you reach the pause at the end of the breath, fling energy out in all directions.

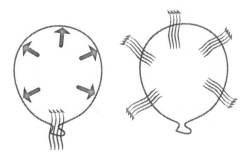

It's like a balloon popping in all directions! Explore how it feels, what directions the energy takes, how far it goes. Put more energy into it and fling the energy out into space.

Where in space are we?

Nowhere special! Maybe a little farther out then we usually go. Most times we fling our energy out without being aware of it. We focus outside ourselves on objects, on projects, on people. We fantasize, building cloud castles somewhere past our head. Some people come out here a lot!

We come out whenever we are struck by art, by beauty. Our mind stills as the beauty of a sunset cuts through the normal static, and we open like a flower to drink it in.

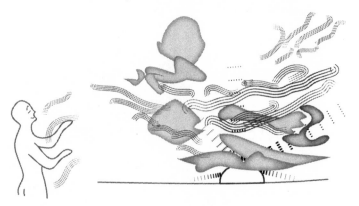

That sounds different, as if the energy is coming in, not going out.

Energy channels run both ways! A work of art is given a great deal of energy by the artist. When we stop in front of it, we can open to it, and share the intent and energy of the artist. The more we open, the clearer the channel. And the more intense and joyful the experience of the art.

It works the same way when we deal with people or with anything. The less static we have in our senses, the clearer the senses become, and the more we perceive and experience.

Try clearing the static from the heart chakra. Expand your chest in a circle as you breathe in. Hold the circle as you breathe out. Breathe in and expand. Breathe out, and fling the circle outwards.

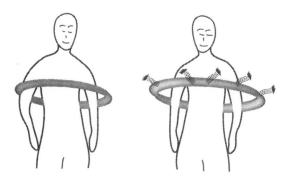

Explore clearing the static from other chakras. Each one will release differently.

It feels odd...

Most of us are accustomed to having static around us all the time. Having static feels normal. When we have too much static, we instinctively release the excess. We play vigorous games, we jump off bridges. We go to amusement parks and take thrilling rides, yelling our heads off, tightening up our bodies to throw off as much energy as possible. It feels great!

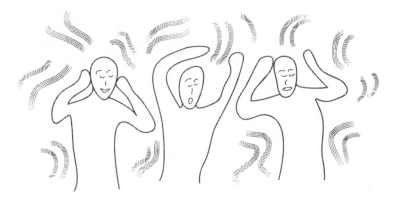

We even use meditation to still our bodies and wait for the static to dissolve.

Clearing the static using our awareness is much faster and more thorough. Once we clear the static, we have a much better channel to the universe.

26 Touching the universe

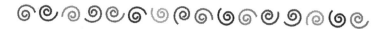

Don't we touch the universe all the time?

Yes, we do. We can't help it. The universe is all around us, IS us. Most of the time, though, we are focused on specific things. We look at furniture and buildings, cars, clothes, food. We touch them, we establish connections to them.

We look at humans, at ideas, at art. We touch them, too.

Don't we touch the universe through spiritual traditions?

Sometimes. That's part of what keeps them going! We try to touch the universe in prayer, in ceremony. In shamanic traditions we may try to touch aspects of the universe such as wind or sky.

We may try to touch the universe through an image. We may try through song and chant, through dance, through meditation.

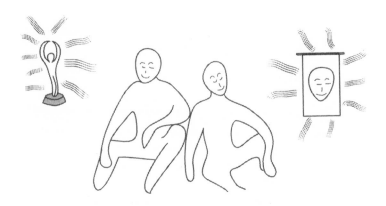

We often try to touch the universe through other humans who have strong energy channels. At least, stronger than ours.

Stronger?

All of us have met or know of teachers, healers or yogis who have a strong connection with the universe. Or shamans, monks or religious people of any tradition. That's what draws us to them.

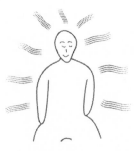

Touching the universe through intermediaries is as old as human history. But you don't need an intermediary to touch the universe directly. You don't need to become a monk or a saint. You just have to tune in once a day.

Once a day?

That's a good place to start. Because at least you can remember to tune in before going to bed! Clear the static, touch the universe, and sleep very well, indeed.

Doesn't it take special training?

It takes basic human wiring, which the universe has provided. We've already done the hard work, by clearing our static. Let's go a little further and see what we see.

Seat yourself comfortably. Breathe in, and breathe down, relaxing and centering.

Expand your head as you breathe in. Release inward on the out-breath. Play with this until it feels comfortable.

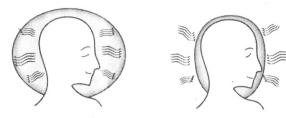

Expand as you breathe in, and hold the expansion as you gently let your breath go. On one of your breaths, expand out and release outward in all directions.

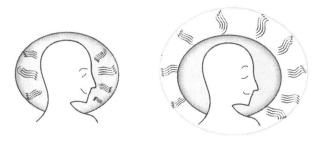

Hold the expansion! You may feel a vacuum in your head. To equalize everything, breathe in with the pelvis. Let your breath flow up through your head.

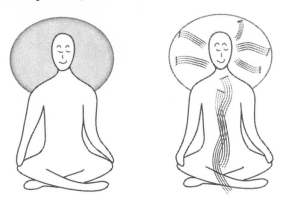

Good! Now we have a clear field to reach out and explore.

Reach where?

Pick a direction. Straight out the front of the head will do. Breathe in, and breathe out through the front of your head. It will feel almost like a narrow balloon extending out in front.

Play with it; see how far you can reach.

When you are ready, pop through the end of the balloon in a straight line.

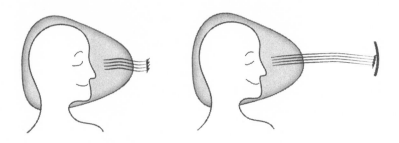

The first time, the line may travel out, and come back in to your head. Play with extending the line. Play with holding it for a longer time. At some point it will dive further and catch like a magnet anchoring to another magnet. It's much like what happens when you find *down*!

With a little practice, you'll be able to hold the line open and steady. Explore further, and you'll even be able to send pulses out, and feel pulses coming back.

Where are we?

Right where we have always been. We've just expanded our balloon, extended our senses. We do this as children, touching things around us, making them familiar. Although we tend to keep our personal energy systems close to home, we can reach out at any time to the universe we live in.

Some traditions make a very big deal of this, surrounding it with lots of hoopla, and providing all kinds of rules. But the universe is always around us. We can reach out at any time and touch it.

Once a day is good.

Where can we go?

Anywhere, really. The funny thing is that as you explore extending your awareness, you will find that you lose the need to go someplace. The more we explore, the more we find that everything is connected. And the more we want to connect.

More?

Think of a space telescope with many movable mirrors. What the telescope can see depends on where the mirrors are focused and on how well they are focused.

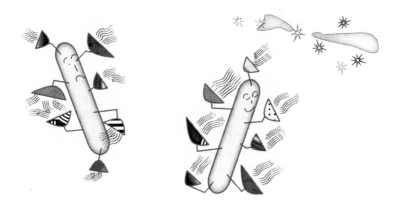

To get a better connection, use more mirrors. You take in more energy that way.

More is better?

Can we have any doubt? We revere humans who have had great connections to the universe. We know that higher states of energy are the way we evolve. We also know that keeping our energy confined and trying to spin in the same circles is a very unsatisfying way to live. The universe is always evolving, so we might as well go along!

So how do we get more?

By exploring. The first step is learning to pop through the balloon, which we have done.

Explore extending out in two directions. Explore diagonals. Explore extending from different chakras or multiple chakras.

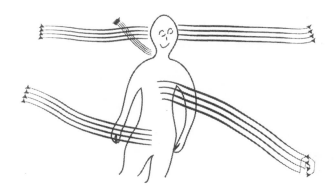

As you increase your awareness and the amount of energy you can handle, you may find that you can fire everything up at once. You can expand in all directions.

The more you extend, the more you can touch. And the more the universe can touch you.

27 Seeking the cells

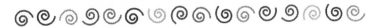

The cells in our body?

Yes. When we are children, we feel with our cells. Children have such an intense experience of the universe. They glow with it. We call it the happiness of a child. And we often share it in watching them, interacting with them.

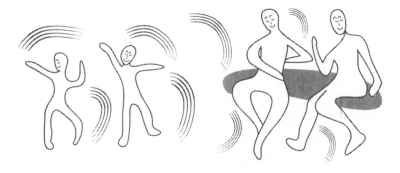

Our cells feel the happiness in theirs, and perk up.

Why in the cells?

Well it's still energy, really, but the cells are a useful reference point. Cells are the basic building blocks of our physical body. You could say that cells are the smallest antenna in our body. They receive and give off energy like any other dissipative system. They receive the energy of the universe and process it on an organic level.

What the cells experience, humans call love. The love we feel in our cells is the cellular expression of the energy of the universe.

Love is in the cells?

Hah! Yes! A very good description. That's why love is so hard to pin down: we feel it everywhere in our body!

It's how we love food, and kittens, though they are not at all the same thing. We love nature, we love the energy of a city, we love driving cars, and we love new clothes. In fact, we can love just about anything, if we can get our cells to go for it.

What happens if they don't?

It's always a losing proposition. We can convince ourselves that we love someone, but if the cells don't agree, we will be eventually left with a pretense, a busted pattern lacking in energy.

We can't, of course, separate our cells from the energy in our body. But it is very useful to consider them a partner in the conversation!

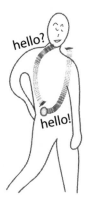

Conversation?

A conversation of desire. Our cells desire food, rest, sleep, exercise, energy, warmth, more food. Have you ever made love to someone where it felt like the cells in your body were making love to theirs? Or read about that kind of desire and yearned for it?

Our cells are all about connecting to the universe. To the desire, the passion, the energy. Even when we deny that such desire could exist, we still feel it.

Why?

A child is created when the energy of the universe in both parents combines. A child grows in a womb, connected by energy to the universe, and to the smaller universe of the mother's body.

The single cell is bathed directly in energy from all sides. As the new life develops more cells, that is no longer the case. Patterns begin to form to transfer the energy from the boundary to the interior.

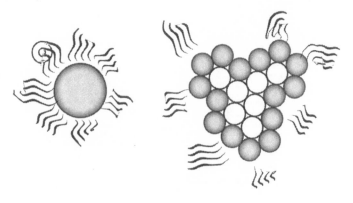

The child grows, and emerges to be a physically separate being. But we never forget the feeling of being bathed directly in the energy of the universe, or in the energy of the womb. It is our first home.

And we try to get back?

That's one way to look at it. Back to the womb, back to the universe. But it is more useful to consider that it is really the connection to the universe we desire. We are here, now. Might as well connect where we are!

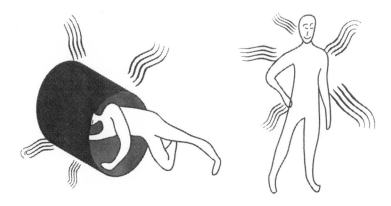

So we wake the cells to love?

A very lovely way to put it. Sometimes it seems that our cells are mostly asleep. They don't start out that way in children. In children cells are always growing, exploring, having to cope with new things, because everything is new.

As children grow, they develop patterns. The patterns channel energy through the body. Posture develops, so does personality. The child begins to rely more on the patterns, less on the individual cells.

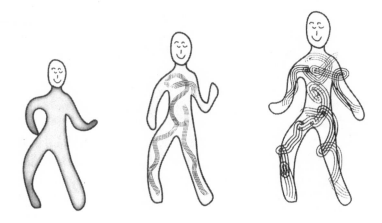

The evolution accelerates in adolescence, when there is intense growth, new wiring, new experiences and new personality traits. The cells are now yearning for direct experience, as energy runs more and more in patterns and less in individual cells.

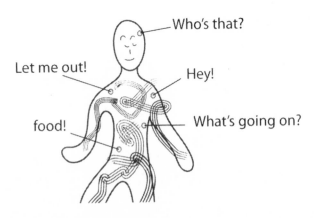

As young adults, adult patterns can seem very confining. We hold on to adolescence and the yearning of the cells. If we run the same patterns over and over, the cells get buried deeper. But they still yearn. So we give them food, we give them pleasure, we give them excitement. What we need to do is give them the energy of the universe.

How?

It's something we do instinctively whenever we feel love for something. We soften with a whole area of our bodies, receiving and sending out energy from our cells.

We can explore this through our arm and leg triangle. Earlier, we released tension in the triangle by releasing a tense position. We can also hold the position and release with our cells in that position.

Seat yourself comfortably. Breathe in, and breathe down. Grab a foot with your hand, and stretch out with a little tension. The exact position doesn't matter.

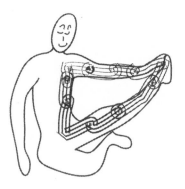

Pause a moment, and look at the triangle formed by your arm, leg, and torso. Run your gaze around the triangle until you can sense the triangle as a whole.

Breathe in, and breathe down, holding the position. Breathe in, hold the position, and breathe out in all directions from the triangle.

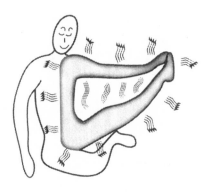

Feel as deeply as you can into the triangle, into your limbs. If you put your awareness into it, your cells are bound to wake up!

Try different positions, different parts of your body. Twist your back a little with some tension. Breathe in, and breathe out in all directions, making your back bigger.

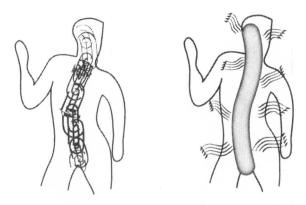

Breathe out from your spine in all directions: front, back, sideways, and up and down. Wake those cells up!

Awake cells feel more love?

Love is an awkward word, because it means so many things. But yes, awake cells feel more of the love, the energy, of the universe.

The pure love that children feel is no myth. It is their cells, which have not yet turned away from the universe to channel energy around the dents, the holes, the bruises of living in the world.

Awareness in the cells is not just for children. Wake up as many of your cells as you can. They will tell you more about love than all the novels, all the poems, in the world.

28 Finding home

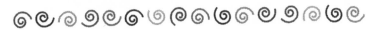

Home?

Home is the universe. It is indisputably our home: we are in it and of it. It is inside us and outside us. How can we not explore?

We've ventured out a little ways, releasing static and expanding our balloon, extending energy out into space. Working from the inside out.

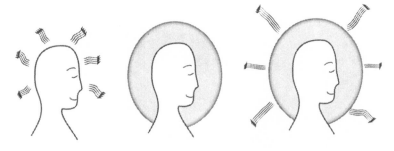

What happens if we simply connect the two?

Connect inside and outside?

It might be more accurate to say, since they are already connected, that we are increasing our awareness of the connection.

We do this by adding, bit by bit, to what we have already learned. We will clear the static from the mind chakra, and throw out some lines. If we throw out enough lines in enough different directions, they will blend into a bigger picture.

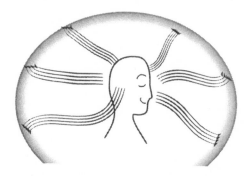

Sit comfortably, breathe in, and breathe down. Clear the static by expanding with your breath and releasing the energy out.

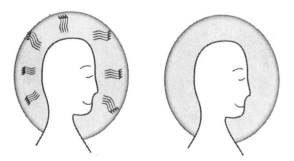

Breathe up your back through the top of your head to equalize the pressure.

Breathe out from the front of your head a couple times, until the front of the balloon gives way. Push it farther, until it makes a connection like two magnets coming together.

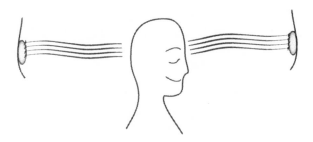

Add another line from your head out the back. You will feel a bit like you are hanging from a clothesline! Use your breath any way you like to adjust.

Add a third line out to the right. And a fourth to the left. Add a line upward, and one downward.

Your awareness will be centered as never before at the point where the lines come together.

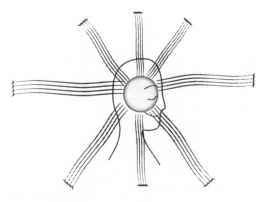

Add a couple diagonal lines. When you feel as though you can't add any more lines, rest a moment.

Feel for the center point where all those lines come together. Breathe in, and let it expand. Breathe in, and let it flow out the lines to their end.

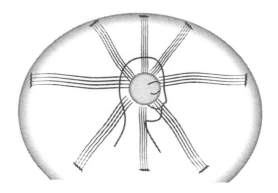

The first time you will scurry back to your head from this unfamiliar territory! But it is only the universe, and you can go back out whenever you like for more exploring.

How much more is there?

An amazing amount. Inside and outside. Just as we have explored in our own bodies finding lines, building them into patterns, and merging patterns into wholes, we do the same in sensing the universe.

When you have enough lines, you will feel like a tree branching out into space. When the tree becomes big enough all around you, you can touch the edge of the universe.

That sounds too big...

It's not nearly big enough! Beyond the edge of the universe is the universe flinging itself outward in all directions.

Being able to sense the universe with awareness is the heritage of humans, and perhaps their very purpose. We've come this far, how about just a little farther?

Seat yourself comfortably, breathe in, and breathe down.

The territory is familiar enough now. Clear the static by releasing your head outward. Send out your lines as far as you can, and as many as are comfortable. Rest and savor the moment.

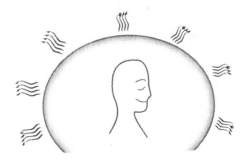

We will release from the outer edge of our lines. Breathe in, expanding to feel the outer edge where the lines end. Move your awareness around from front to back, top to bottom. This is your current balloon.

Breathe in, expanding and pushing a little on the outer edge. Play with the edge a bit.

Breathe in, and fling yourself outward.

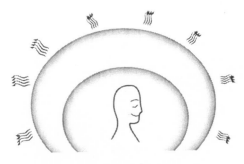

If you can, rest a moment on this new outer edge. If you can't, drop back, rest a moment, and then come back out to the edge.

From this point outward is the onrushing of the universe. Touch it for yourself. Release outward and feel the extraordinary passion, a passion we recognize in every cell and every space of our bodies.

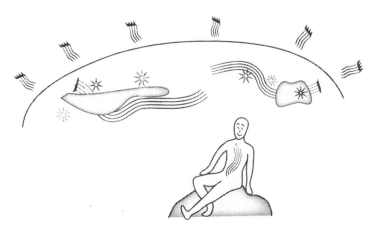

This is far past the realm of words, or even images. Beyond what the mind alone can handle. In fact, it takes a whole colony of cells!

If it doesn't seem believable, go back and explore for yourself. Do you have something better to do in this existence?

29 The dance of Shiva/Shakti

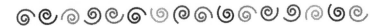

A dance?

A useful way to look at the flow of the universe. Humans have created an astonishing variety of ways to look at the universe in thought, words, dance, music, emotions. Religion and philosophy have morphed over and over as human culture has evolved.

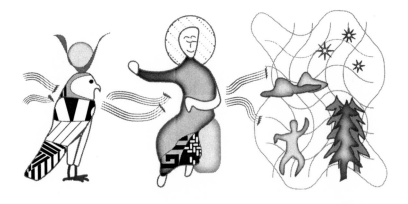

Many traditions have focused on creation/destruction, order/chaos. But in the universe, science confirms that energy can neither be created nor destroyed, only changed or moved.

The universe is always evolving. The patterns and structures change, and grow more complex. As the universe evolves, the changes in energy flow are not light/dark, life/

death, good/bad. The energy flow is much better described as push/pull, or outward/inward. In other words, shiva/shakti.

That's the way we feel it: a confusing and delicious flow of male/female, outward/inward, push/pull.

Push/pull?

Our lives are full of pushing and pulling! We pull in food, thoughts, emotions, culture. We push out emotions, thoughts, innovations.

We push out into our lives, into society. And we get pulled into all kinds of situations and predicaments.

Relationships are full of pushing and pulling. You could define an excellent relationship as an excellent pushing and pulling between two people!

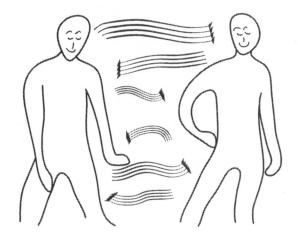

Shiva/shakti is more than pushing and pulling, though. Shiva/shakti is also outside and inside: we push outwards and pull inwards.

So, too, in the universe. Shiva is the universe pushing out, expanding in all directions, yelling her head off on the greatest roller coaster of all time. Shakti is the encompassing and evolving of her expanding space.

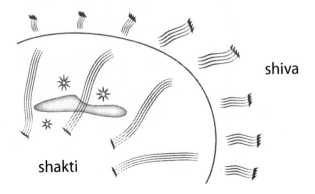

We feel both in our bodies. Often, we work mostly with one or the other. When we connect with other humans, it's often shiva to shiva, shiva to shakti, shakti to shiva, and shakti to shakti.

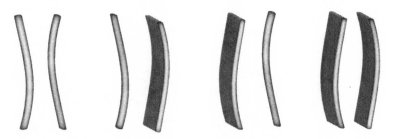

We can also combine them.

Combine them?

Combine the energies and combine the perspectives. Shiva/shakti is push/pull, expand/encompass, and is also looking out and looking in. Let's combine the energies first. Sit comfortably, breathe in, and breathe down.

Breathe in a few times up the front shiva channel from your pelvis. Expand the chakras on the front channel. Reach for the shakti channel behind it, feeling for the creases of your hips and of your shoulders. Breathe a few times up the shakti channel until it expands.

Breathe up the back channel. Start at the base and arc up and outside the back to the crown. When you have a feel for the back channel, breathe in along the whole channel. Breathe out, and let the channel expand.

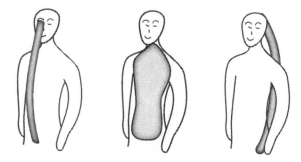

Feel for all three channels. Like we did when we combined our head and knee, let the boundaries of the channels relax and become one boundary.

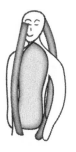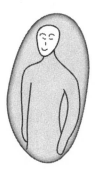

Combining them feels quite different than holding them separately. Now that we can feel both energies, let's explore the different perspectives of shakti/shiva.

Let's use the mind chakra to explore.

Use your breath to expand your mind in all directions. See how far you can go.

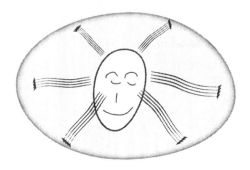

Feel the far edge of your expansion. Fill up the space until your boundary is the far edge. Look outwards.

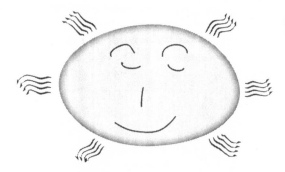

This is shiva, pushing out.

Turn around on the edge and look inward to the center. It will feel much like it did when we centered our awareness with many different lines in all directions. Only this time we're looking in from the outside!

This is shakti, encompassing the center.

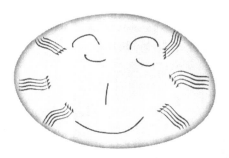

My head feels very large...

Try some of the other chakras to balance things out. Try the heart chakra. Feel from the center as far out around you as you can. Feel from the edge back into the center.

You will know without question when you do it. The body responds instantly to such changes of perspective and energy flow. Feeling shiva and shakti is to feel the tension, the passion, of the universe.

And, of course, everyone feels it differently!

Why?

When we looked at dissipative structures we saw that evolution means jumping from one level of complexity to another. Increasing the energy as you go. If every element in the system is complex, the complexity is that much greater, and butterfly points occur faster.

Having a unique pattern of shiva/shakti in every human raises enormously the complexity of the human species. More ways to interact, faster learning of new behaviors. Faster evolution.

Add sexual reproduction and environmental stress, two
of the best tools for evolving a species. Sexual reproduction
keeps changing the genetic mix. Environmental stress changes
the behavior patterns. Individual experiences re-wire basic
patterns and create new ones.

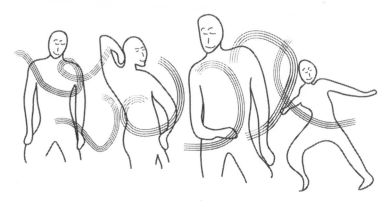

Our evolutionary picture is now a dance, a weaving,
of many elements. Of shakti/shiva, sexual reproduction,
environmental change, order, chaos and butterfly points. Of
individual experience and choices adding flavors and nuance.

Enough strands to see the larger fabric.

30 The great experiment

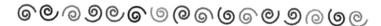

Experiment?

That's the way science would describe it. An experiment is trying something out to see what happens. What would happen if you mix lots of elements together and stir through time?

To the universe, it would be called evolution. A creation. A pattern in the larger fabric of the expansion and evolution of the universe.

What kind of experiment?

The same kind we do as children. Have you ever played with dolls or toy soldiers? You move them here and there. You wish they could talk back, so you invent words for them to say.

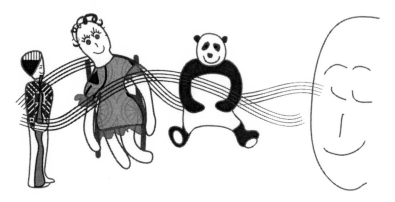

We think how nice it would be if our playmates could act on their own, talk back to us of their own accord, have a real conversation.

What we as humans cannot do, the universe can and does.

We're *playmates*?

Hah! Yes! Playing in the only game in town. Playing with the universe.

No one who has felt shakti/shiva can imagine that it is only a game. No matter how playful the universe can be! The universe is passionately rushing outward, evolving in all directions. Humans are sharing in that evolution.

The universe evolved a star and a planet that would give her the conditions she needed. Gave it a single large moon to keep the energy moving in a certain way.

She played with the building blocks of life, developed DNA as a code that could replicate and hold patterns. She created cells, gave them motion, increased the complexity in the ways they acquired and used energy. Grew them into organisms.

She hit a couple of unpromising leads, wiped the slate clean, and started over.

Started over?

Life has nearly been extinguished on earth at least twice. Geologists have read the pattern in ancient rocks.

There have also been several mass extinctions of species in earth's history. You could say that all species have been extinguished except for the ones living today!

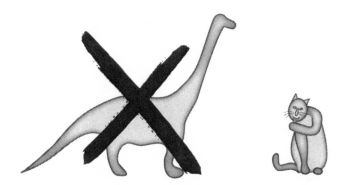

The experiment comes to an end for more than 99% of all species. The universe perfected reptilian wiring and explored new avenues in dinosaurs. They didn't work out. The goddess learned what size of animal was too big. And what amount of complexity was not enough.

Every lesson learned was put to use. To the reptile brain she added a mammalian brain and wiring. She took what dinosaurs knew of herd behavior, of aggression. She wove it into new patterns, whole new behaviors, increased complexity.

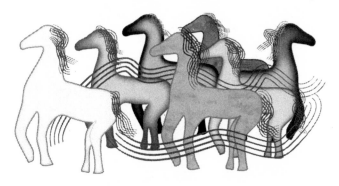

She created a new brain, a new weave, for primates, exploring tribal behavior, curiosity. New patterns for child-rearing, sex, bonding, and using tools.

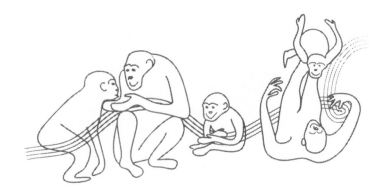

Then she was ready to start humans.

Everything leads to humans?

Only if you focus on humans. The entire earth is alive with the energy of the universe. It sings its own song, tones documented in human songs, poetry and cultural traditions. The songs of whales still baffle us. We know they sing to the universe all around them. We don't yet know what they are saying.

Humans may be partners of the goddess, but so is everything else!

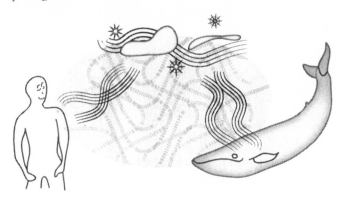

Okay. Back to humans...

The common ancestor of chimpanzees and humans had the right mix to continue. Humans and chimps share 95% of their genes. But humans have a bigger processor, and different genes turned on.

For humans she increased the size of the primate brain. Several times. In different human species.

She gave us the desire to explore the universe. No species has ever wandered as far of their own accord as humans. We even want to reach the stars!

As climates changed, the new conditions created new wiring. Dinosaurs could not survive climate change, but humans had the tools to innovate and survive.

She fine-tuned the amount of aggression, but by then the woolly mammoths and the sabre-toothed tigers had been hunted to extinction. Left as memories on cave walls.

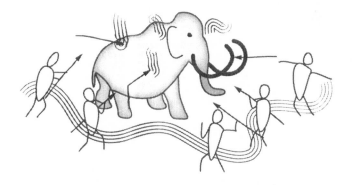

The species grew, developing language far more than our brother chimps. We developed stories about how we experience the world. And ceremonies that explored our connection to the universe.

This all took a long time...

A very long time. Most of human history, in fact. We look back in amazement now that so much has happened in such a short period of time, these last few millennia.

The time frame makes sense when you look at the evolution of dissipative structures. An open system takes in energy, and jumps to a higher level. The rate of jumping accelerates over time, as does the amount of complexity.

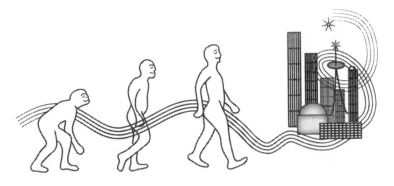

It may be that the amount of time it has taken humans to evolve is the minimum necessary for the universe to accomplish the evolution. There was a great deal of weaving and reweaving to do.

Weaving and reweaving?

Humans were organized into family groupings and tribes that wandered all over the world. In many places at roughly the same time humans settled down and started farming. A reweaving, a few genes turned on, or off.

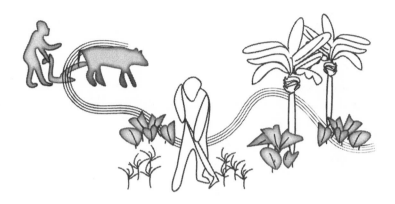

In the agricultural period tradition became culture. A quantum leap in complexity and organized energy.

Anthropologist Jared Diamond in *Guns, Germs and Steel* showed how the availability of resources, of energy, caused some groups of humans to develop civilizations quickly. Other groups of humans developed more slowly. Or remained in the Stone Age.

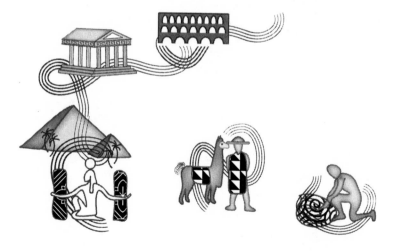

If we look at energy flow, we see constant flow and change in the great, east-west highway of Asia. Famine, war, trade, animals, disease. Writing developed. Culture became civilization.

In other places, the energy flows were more isolated, more limited. Central and South America created empires that lasted, but did not evolve as quickly. Sub-Saharan Africa evolved empires that the environment could not sustain.

The Pacific created interesting island cultures, different from the continents. Australia, parched of resources, barely kept alive a tribal culture. The Stone Age experience was refined over millennia into the rich concepts we call *aboriginal dreamtime*.

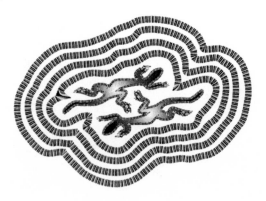

Different energy flows in different cultures...

We can think of them as energy systems composed of humans, interacting with each other. Look at the ebb and flow of history to see religions, ideas, fashions, tools spinning, expanding, being swept away.

In Egypt a focus on the afterlife. In China a focus on the family. In Europe a focus on the individual. Swirl cultures together through trade, war, migration. Send the barbarians to break things up and inject new energy, new genes.

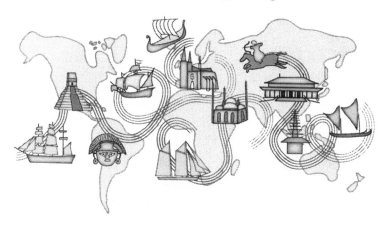

Send in new ideas. That the universe is not alive. That science can discover truths and improve life. Spur humans to feel more empowered. Let them discover the universe on their own. One discovery will lead to the next.

Discoveries have come quickly in recent times. Gone is the notion of eternity. Gone is the independent observer. Gone is the notion that matter and energy are different. Gone is the notion that random chance by itself could possibly have created the world.

What we've found is a universe both expanding and evolving. And evolving humans to be individual, separate, and capable of connecting back to her.

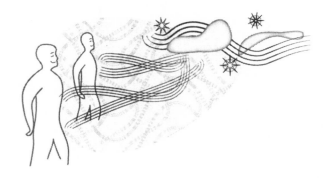

Why not just use better wiring?

There isn't any! People used to think that the universe was eternal, and planned everything out. We know differently. Even given the possibilities of multi-verses, eleven dimensions, bounce theory, and cosmic string theory, the universe was born, and is rushing through space and time. The universe creates as it goes along.

Humans, too. We create as we go along, inventing new forms to express our growing awareness.

When we look at a leaf, we see the color, the shape, the way it moves in the wind, the way it opens to the sun. We see the cells absorbing the sunlight. Converting energy into plant.

We see the leaf and plant as part of a much larger ecology with many species, many energy flows. We see the ecology as one flow in a global energy system.

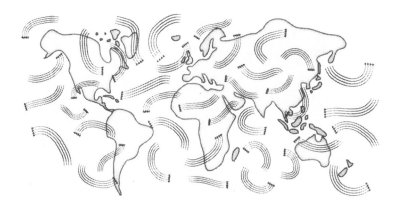

We make our awareness of patterns both wide and deep, just as the universe does. We continually enhance our wiring with new perspectives and energy flows. We have the best wiring we are able to create.

31 Creating wiring

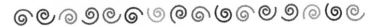

How do you create wiring?

Our environment is always moving/changing through time, providing new energy. On the basic energy template of our DNA we swirl together the energy of cultural influences and direct personal experience.

We can choose at any butterfly point to run the energy through existing channels. We can choose to adjust our wiring to handle the new energy. We can even choose to create new wiring ourselves through exploring.

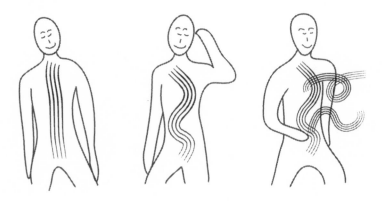

Exploring how?

Just as we have all along, using our awareness to look inside and outside our bodies. Using the mirrors of our chakras to look around, and look at each other.

Each other?

It's only a step past connecting them. Let's use the heart and mind.

Breathe in, and breathe down, centering. Open your heart with your breath front and back. Bring your awareness back into your mind and breathe your mind open front and back.

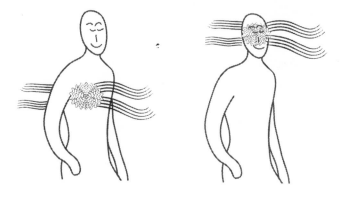

Use the front of your open mind to gaze at your heart. Go to the front of your open heart and gaze at your mind. With both circuits in your awareness, the two flows will become one circuit.

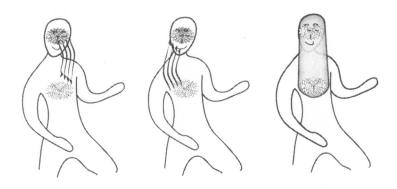

It's like an expanding ring of light...

Of energy, yes. Opening your chakras to each other produces a wonderful floating feeling. And improves the connection between them.

We can build new connections, too. We can travel out to a new spot to reach farther. If a man fishes from the end of a dock, his line can only go so far into the lake. If he travels out in a boat, he can reach much farther.

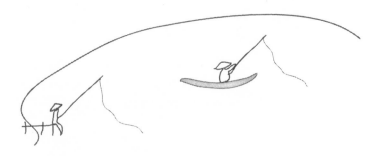

Let's see if we can create a boat, a new wiring spot. Or at least visualize how we might do it.

Seat your self comfortably, breathe in, and breathe down.

Expand your head with your breath in different directions until it feels nice and open. Breathe in, and breathe out through the front of your head. Cast a line straight out until it catches. Use your breath to settle into a comfortable position.

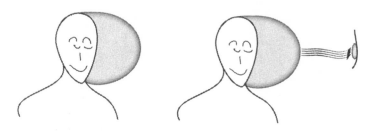

Send some energy out the line to the end. Let the end expand into a glowing ball as you breathe a couple times..

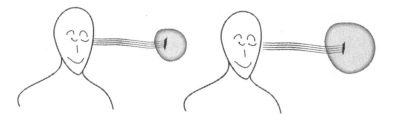

Cast the line past the ball. If you can, go to the ball itself and cast out from there.

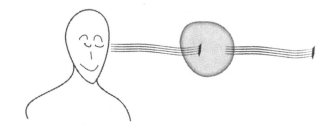

Like casting out from a boat. Or a personal spaceship!

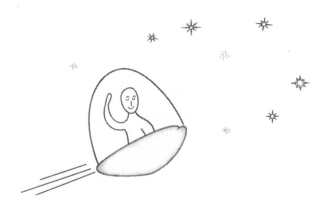

Images can take us a long way. What we are actually doing is weaving energy, creating new wiring. To add to the cultural wiring we are also creating.

Creating cultural wiring...

Previous cultures gave us the wiring to create the current one, our first attempt at a global culture. A new flow of energy, ideas, images, genes.

Ideas move at the speed of light through optical cables, through the Internet. Wiring humans together in new ways. Creating a culture that stretches from reggae to the Taj Mahal, the latest cell phone to fusion cuisine.

The new global culture is confusing...

It may well seem chaotic and dysfunctional. Humans needed enough shiva energy to not only reach the top of the food chain, but to keep going and fling humans and satellites into space.

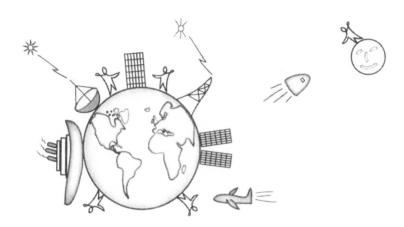

Shiva energy expressed in human aggressiveness has made for some dark times. For individuals. For cultures. Trauma that puts dents in us definitely gets our attention!

Looking also at the accomplishments suggests that Shiva/ Shakti is balanced in humans the same way it is balanced in the universe. And humans are getting better at channeling shiva energy away from the basic wiring of aggression. Into forward, more productive pursuits.

There are more humans alive on the earth today than in all of human history combined. Exchanging energy in complex, new ways. Getting closer as individuals and as a culture to the universe. We just have to keep improving the wiring!

And then?

There is no then that makes sense in the human scale. We simply keep evolving with the universe, part of her evolution, and a rich weaving in her fabric.

That's what makes it such a great adventure! It's an open-ended game, and we get to play.

It's hard to believe.

No belief is necessary. Explore it for yourself!

32 The art of exploring

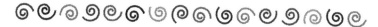

Exploring is an art?

Tantra is artful exploration of the universe. Free-form encompassing, moment by moment. It is directed forward, outward, inward. Every human creates a unique art of exploring.

What do you take with you? What do you pack for the journey?

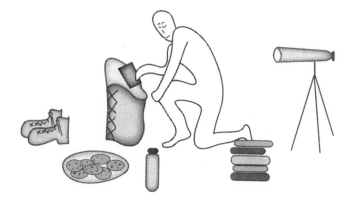

Everything you have?

Of course! Take your body. Notice how your body moves, your posture, your habits. Where is the tension? How do you release it? Where does it hurt? How do you compensate?

Take the body wiring. What makes you jumpy, what makes you relaxed, what makes you stiffen? What tickles?

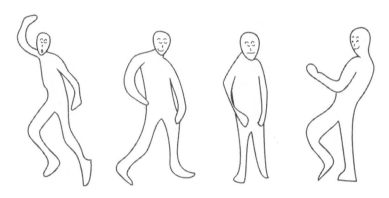

What energy centers do you use the most? Which ones feel closed up? The heart? The second chakra? The base chakra?

Take the ground. Breathe and find *down*.

Take your mind. What patterns is it running? What thoughts keep coming back and coming back? From what thoughts do you shy away? What do you push aside?

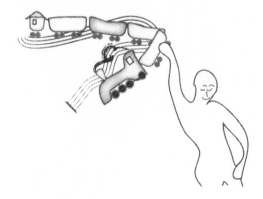

Take your energy.

How are you using your energy? What gives you more energy? What takes it away? When do you open up? When do you close?

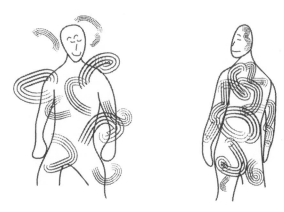

Take your attention. Do you know where it is? What it is doing? Do you try to split it among several things? Do you focus on only one thing at a time? Can you do both?

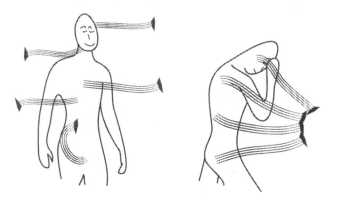

Both?

Try both sides of the road. Try the middle.

One of Buddha's great insights was the value of the middle way, moderation. Not going so far in any one direction that you twist all your patterns around it.

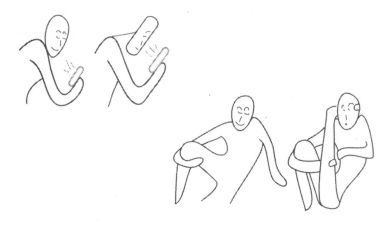

The middle path doesn't mean staying only in the middle, it means covering the whole road without falling over the edge. Doing everything in moderation, including excess!

How do we find the middle path?

With awareness. If we pay exquisite attention to what we are doing, we can consciously choose how to respond at each next moment. We can avoid going over the edge.

In the film *Baraka* by Ron Fricke, there is a scene on a busy Japanese street. Fashionable shoppers hurry to and fro, but the camera follows a monk, dressed traditionally and carrying a bell. With each ring of the bell, the monk takes one gracefully careful step.

The monk is tuned to a completely different rhythm of energy frequencies than everyone else around him. He *chooses* it so.

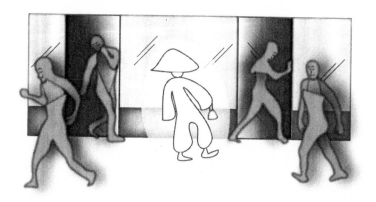

So, too, we can choose in any moment our action. Monk or shopper. In our modern world, we must be many things, so we shift from monk to shopper and back whenever we need to.

Travelling through life is no different than travelling to a new place, because every moment is new. At every moment, every butterfly point, we choose our action.

We can choose to notice. We can choose to move. We can choose to flex. We can choose to step up.

Whoa! One at a time!

To notice something is to focus our attention on it, however briefly. When you go to a new place, you notice a lot. You notice the light, the colors, the textures, the different architecture and the swirl of energy.

We notice one thing, then another. Our eyes open wider to notice as many things as we can. Like a child's face enjoying fireworks for the first time.

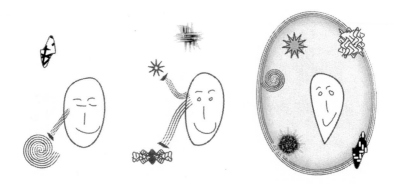

Taking exquisite notice of things is one of the sharpest pleasures in life, no matter where you are.

Take exquisite notice of how you respond to others. How they respond to you. How do they *not* respond? What do they *not* do or say?

What people do not do or say, what they do not stretch forth to you, is every bit as interesting. And tells you more about their boundaries than anything they put into words.

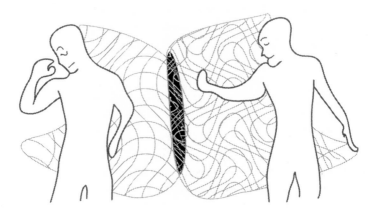

We often don't pay attention to how the boundaries between two people interact. We just run our standard patterns at each other.

Standard patterns?

Our cultural and personal knowledge, our assumptions, guide us through our own patterns, and find what we assume are the appropriate responses to the other person's patterns. Our awareness checks in every couple sentences to make sure everything is on track.

But we can focus our attention. On anything we choose.

If we like, we can turn our full attention on another human. We can read every flow of energy and create a new response every time. Throw the energy. Bounce the energy. Reflect it back. Incorporate it and send back something new.

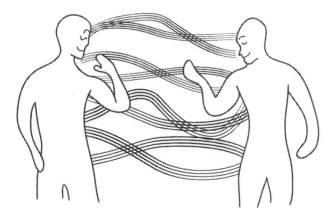

If the other person is also paying full attention the flows mix, they entwine, they merge. It's exquisite. Especially if you keep moving.

Moving...

Move your body in different ways. Move your awareness to different points around your body. Move your awareness to your whole body. Move your awareness from the physical body to the chakras.

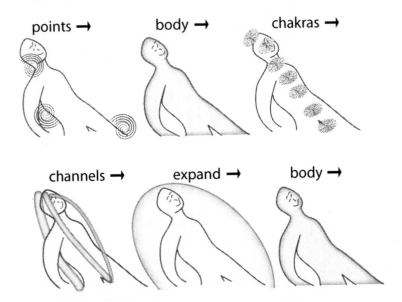

Move your awareness from the chakras to the shiva/shakti channels. To the back channel. To the universe. Back to your body.

Don't get stuck anywhere!

Stuck?

Some traditions place a high emphasis on various energy states. So do drug-users.

Energy states?

In most of our exercises we've released tension and increased the amount of energy flowing through the body. As you work deeper and loosen up more channels, the flowing energy in the system increases and moves faster. It is often enough to tip the system into ecstasy.

What *is* ecstasy?

It's a powerful excitation of your energy system that is more than the channels can handle. The channels vibrate and expand to accommodate the increased energy. Expanded too often, or expanded too far, the channels burn out, at least for a while.

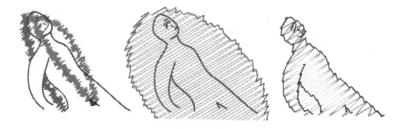

We see the extremes in trauma cases and drug addicts, but any too-excited channels burn out over time.

How do we avoid burn-out?

By flexing and expanding our boundaries rather than trying to break them.

Play with the boundaries of your awareness. Push out from them in one direction, then the other. Try to go in both directions at once.

Switch the left and right boundaries of your awareness.
Switch the top and bottom, front and back, inside and outside.

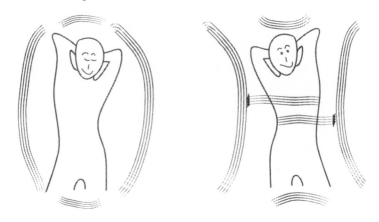

Move your awareness outside your body. Try going to the
outer edge of your awareness and looking back. Your body
will react instantly to the change in perspective. What does it
do?

Try to look out the back of each chakra!

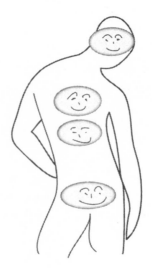

This is disorienting!

Yes, as you venture farther out, you can feel disoriented, electric, overwhelmed, even. That's when you can step up.

Step up?

As good a term as any to describe the action. It *feels* like stepping-up, just as you step-up to respond to any situation. Stepping up to the counter in a store, stepping up to express your self, stepping up to volunteer.

When the motion seems great, step up to encompass it and find stillness.

When things seems chaotic, step up to see the larger pattern in which the chaos makes sense.

When tension makes you want to shrink back, make yourself larger than it, and find the flow.

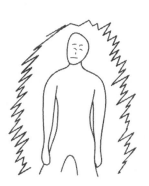 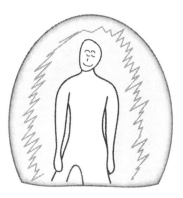

Stepping up is a great tool for explorers. Stepping up is saying *Yes* to the evolving universe... the only game in town!

33 A final cup of tea

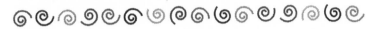

Do we empty out our assumptions again?

Yes! At least temporarily.

We can't really live in the world without assumptions. They are an indispensable tool for navigation. They are not bedrock, though. The universe is. And the universe is changing at every moment, evolving new surprises that will not match our assumptions.

So empty out your assumptions as often as you can, and look at the world afresh!

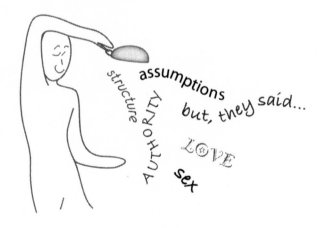

You didn't talk much about sex...

Didn't need to. If you can notice your body and energy channels, and notice your partner's body and energy channels, you will discover a richness that no mere technique can ever approach. Not just in sex, but in everything.

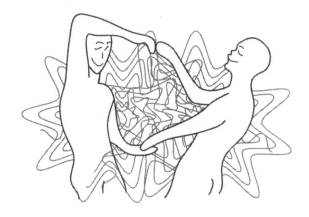

Sexual patterns whether boring or kinked are a reaching out of sexual energy in a limited pattern. It is a search for responses in others that will link to our own pattern.

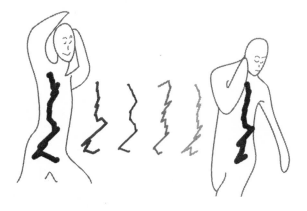

If instead you unfold your energy patterns and use your awareness, you begin working on broadband.

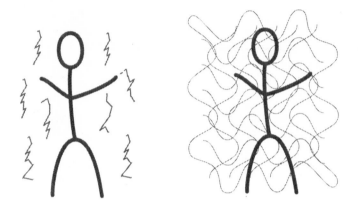

Sexual energy still seems different, somehow.

That's because sexual energies are not broadband. They are a set of frequencies in the second chakra energies of desire and passion. They feel especially good because humans are wired so well for them.

Desire and passion can power anything. When channeled specifically through the frequencies of sex, they power discovery, ecstasy, and the creation of new humans.

What about love?

The thing everyone is looking for? Love is the word we use for the energies of the heart chakra. That everyone is searching for love tells us that we hold our heart energies too close.

Many, many teachers have told us to open our hearts. The heart is part of the larger energy flow of our system, touching many patterns. We use this linking to other patterns to think about opening the heart, to sing the heart open, to use the ecstatic pattern of sex to flood the heart with energy.

We use word-drugs to coax our hearts open, and to convince our selves that our hearts *are* open.

We should also work directly with the heart to get the energies we need. Just breathe in and breathe out.

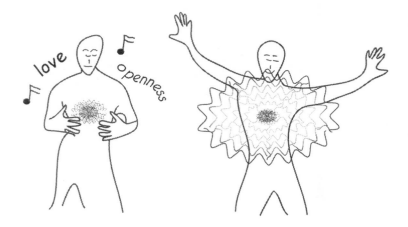

So simple...

Scientists often say that the best answers to be found in the universe are elegantly simple. So don't worry about the words, and the philosophies, and the beliefs. Just straighten out your own energy system. The rewards are beyond our best imagination.

Thank you...

You're very welcome. And thank you, too, and to all the bright bits of the universe in humans, lighting a path that

connects us to the mind, heart, movement, and passion of the
universe.

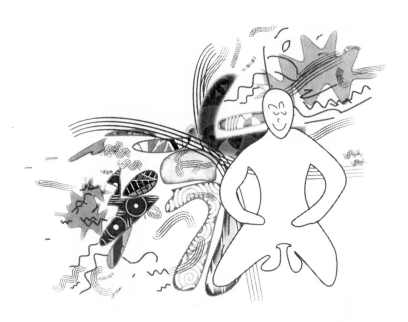

Some interesting explorations

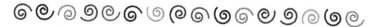

Ilya Prigogine

From Being to Becoming: Time and complexity in the physical sciences

with Isabel Stengers

Order out of Chaos: Man's new dialogue with nature

Prigogine's own explanation of the paradigm of dissipative structures. At times, it's heavy going. Still, no one explains the concepts as well.

Erich Jantsch

The self-organizing universe: Scientific and human implications of the emerging paradigm of evolution

Jantsch's stunning leap in applying the paradigm of dissipative structures.

Daniel Odier

Tantric Quest: An Encounter with Absolute Love

Desire: The Tantric Path to Awakening

Yoga Spandakarika: The Sacred Texts at the Origin of Tantra

Daniel Odier's stories, understandings, and translations of Tantra are more direct than just about anything else written. Like Zen koans, encompass one couplet of the Yoga Spandakarika and you will encompass them all.

Eric D. Schneider & Dorion Sagan

Into The Cool: Energy Flow, Thermodynamics and Life

A well-written, comprehensive overview of all of the major developments of thermodynamic theory, plus interesting speculations.

Georg Feuerstein

Tantra: The Path of Ecstasy

An excellent description of the original cultural traditions of Indian Tantra (one of three streams of Tantra, along with Tibetan Tantra and Kashmiri Shaivism). Shows brilliantly how great insight can be beaten into esoteric submission.

Jared Diamond

Guns, Germs and Steel

A masterful exploration of the energies that have shaped human history.

The film *Baraka*, a Ron Fricke film

> *A beautiful film that illustrates the movement of energy in our world.*

Geoffrey Samuel

> *The Origins of Yoga and Tantra: Indic Religions to the Thirteenth Century*

> *A fascinating study of how historical Tantra came to be so many things to so many different peoples.*

Paul Reps and Nyogen Senzaki, compilers

> *Zen Flesh, Zen Bones: a collection of Zen and Pre-Zen writings*

> *Stories from five centuries of Zen masters. Living in expanded and down to earth states has been around a long time!*

Science Daily web site

> *www.ScienceDaily.com*

> *A digest of news from the expanding edge of science that shows that the world is more complex and moves faster than anyone thought!*

Everything, everywhere...

Contact

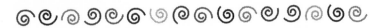

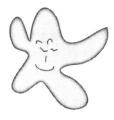

Paul Squassoni has taught tantra yoga for the past several years at Kalani Oceanside Retreat on the Big Island of Hawai`i.

He can be reached through the web site
www.SexandQuantumPhysics.com

Aloha a hui hou!

SEX and QUANTUM PHYSICS
Vol 2: Living in eleven dimensions

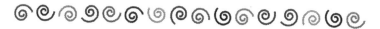

A topic from Volume 2

Did you know the universe has eleven dimensions?!

Over a hundred years ago Albert Einstein proposed that matter and energy were related. Ever since, scientists have explored the boundaries between matter and energy. We have pictured the universe as having four space-time dimensions that curve and twist with gravity. We know that matter is made of complex processes of energy. That the speed of light is the fastest speed in space-time.

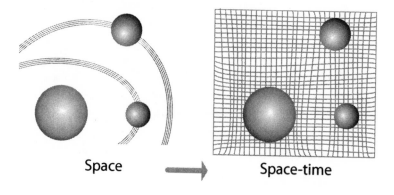

Space ⟶ Space-time

With the development of quantum physics, we discovered more and more about matter and energy. We learned that particles and waves are two different ways of seeing the same energy process. That past the depth of particles and waves lies a quantum foam of probabilities.

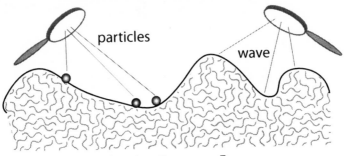

vibrating Quantum Foam

How did we get here?

Science progresses by describing the world as accurately as possible, and then looking for where the description does not fit. For example, if Newton's Law of Gravity describes 99% of what we observe, and Einstein's Laws of Relativity describe 99.5% of what we observe, there is still something left unexplained. What is left over might be the unexplained relationship of gravity and electromagnetism, or a set of quantum circumstances in which the mathematics goes crazy and yields nonsensical results called *quantum anomalies*.

In the case of gravity and electromagnetism, Kaluza-Klein theory shows that Einstein's gravity and Maxwell's electromagnetism are better explained and are unified if you work in five dimensions rather than four. Klein proposed that we cannot see the fifth dimension because it is curled up very small around every point in three-dimensional space.

To show this in a two-dimensional drawing, we shall have to imagine that the grid representing space-time is actually four dimensions.

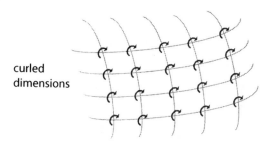

curled
dimensions

While this may seem fanciful, remember that even electricity seemed fanciful only a few hundred years ago. Maxwell's equations of electromagnetism came in 1854, roughly five million years after humans got started!

The more closely physics looked at points in space, the more quantum particles they found, and the more complicated the picture became. To account for all the variations of quantum particles, physicists proposed that the points vibrated like strings sticking out of space-time.

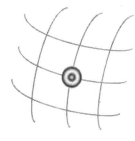

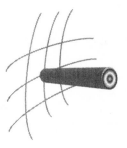

point in space-time
(view from the front)

string in more dimensions
(view from the back)

In fact, to get all the possibilities for all of the particles that may exist, strings must have ten dimensions of space and one of time. It is precisely at eleven dimensions that quantum anomalies (problems in the math) disappear. That would suggest strongly that eleven dimensions is the right number of dimensions for describing the behavior of quantum particles. And quantum particles make up everything else.

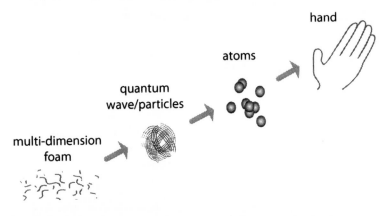

Quantum physics even knows the shape of the interaction between the other seven dimensions and the four dimensions of space-time. The shape is known as a Calabi-Yau manifold, a six-dimensional folded shape with twisting, multi-dimensional holes in it.*

There is a Calabi-Yau shape for every point of space-time.

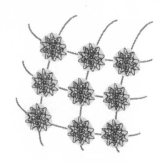

As Shing-Tung Yau puts it in *The Shape of Inner Space*,

> Denizens of the four dimensional realm like us can't ever see this six-dimensional realm, but it's always there, attached to every point in our space. We're just too big to go inside and look around.

This is a very interesting idea! We can imagine that for every point of space-time inside and outside us, there is a six-dimensional knot of energy that gives shape to the four dimensions we *can* see.

To put it another way, the picture that quantum physics has discovered is of space-time being woven by seven other dimensions.

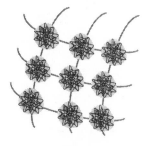

**space-time front
of Calabi-Yau**

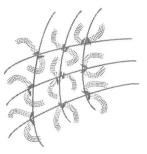

**7-dimension back
of Calabi-Yau**

Oddly enough, this is in perfect accord with the spiritual traditions of humans. Buddhism sees space-time as a veil of illusion. Hinduism sees a pure *atman* beyond space-time. Plato saw a world of ideal forms beyond the mundane appearance of daily life. The Judeo-Christian-Islamic tradition sees space-time as the unfolding of a Creator.

Tantra sees a universe weaving itself.

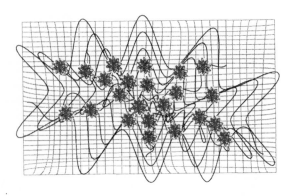

Let's explore that weave a little.

We know that humans are the most complex, unpredictable, and sophisticated energy patterns on our planet. Science has discovered mathematical laws about almost everything except humans. Humans have so many variables and so many complex interactions that to develop equations about humans has proven impossible.

We also know that humans have experienced for their entire history a set of energies that science has never been able to identify in space-time: emotion, desire, intellect. And that we associate these different energies with different parts of the body: heart, loins, head.

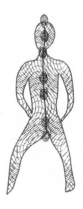

7. crown chakra
6. mind chakra
5. throat chakra

4. heart chakra
3. breath chakra

2. desire chakra
1. base chakra

Tantric Yogi Tells All led us on an exploration of the seven energy centers, or chakras. If quantum physics tells us that seven dimensions of energy are creating space-time**, the correspondence between the seven dimensions and the seven chakras is hard to miss. It seems unlikely that humans would have evolved in such a way as to ignore seven dimensions of the universe's energy! And, in fact, we haven't.

Quantum physics shows us that the basic elements of human nature arise from an eleven-dimension waveform. Human experience has always told us that there are energies and dimensions to the world that we do not see. There's a good possibility that sex and quantum physics have a great deal to say to each other!

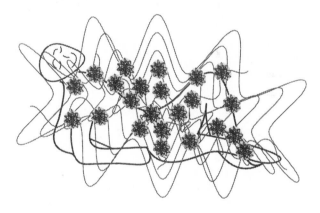

Notes:

*Calabi-Yau manifolds have six dimensions, which when combined with space-time, adds up to ten dimensions. The mathematics for eleven dimensions is so complex that it is largely undeveloped, so physicists reduce the eleven dimensions to ten, and then use Calabi-Yau manifolds in the description.

** This doesn't necessarily violate either the Law of Conservation of Energy or the calculations of total entropy/information in the universe. Some physicists have proposed that the other seven dimensions absorb energy from space-time, weakening the effects of the gravitational force. This would, indeed, make space-time the open, dissipative energy structure suggested by Erich Jantsch, one with energy/information balanced between streaming into, and streaming out of, space-time.

Good Reading...

Brian Greene

> *The Fabric of the Cosmos*
> *The Hidden Reality*

> Greene enthusiastically explains the frontiers of quantum physics as well as anyone.

Shing-Tung Yau and Steve Nadis

> *The Shape of Inner Space*

> A terrific exploration of string theory and geometry from the perspective of the man who proved the existence of Calabi-Yau manifolds.